PUBLIC HEALTH SERVICE OFFICER'S GUIDE

Protocol &

Service Standards

The U.S. Public Health Service Mission

*Protecting, promoting, and advancing
the health and safety of the Nation*

INAUGURAL EDITION

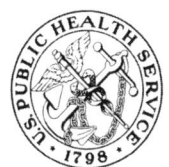

PUBLIC HEALTH SERVICE OFFICER'S GUIDE

❏❏❏❏❏

Protocol &
Service Standards

CAPT James E. Knoben (Ret.)
CDR Alice D. Knoben

U.S. PUBLIC HEALTH SERVICE

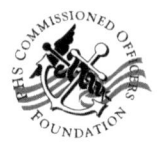

Copyright © 2006 by the

PHS Commissioned Officers Foundation
for the Advancement of Public Health

All rights reserved. No part of this book may be reproduced,
transmitted, or utilized in any form or by any means,
including any information storage and retrieval system,
without written permission from the copyright holder.

The authors have written this book in their private capacity. The views
expressed are those of the authors and do not necessarily represent official
positions of the Office of the Surgeon General, U.S. Public Health Service,
and/or the Department of Health and Human Services.

FIRST EDITION

ISBN 0-9773149-1-X

Exclusive distribution by the

Commissioned Officers Association of the U.S. Public Health Service
8201 Corporate Drive, Suite 200
Landover, Maryland 20797

Printed in the United States of America

CONTENTS

	Foreword	ix
	Preface	xi
	Acknowledgments	xiii

SECTION I.	Uniformed Service Basics 1	
	Protocol and Tradition	1
	Officership	2
	Leadership	4
	Personnel, Ranks and Insignia	7
	Uniform and Device Standards	15

SECTION II.	Military Courtesy & Protocol 29	
	Address & Greeting	29
	Coming to Attention	32
	Flag Etiquette	33
	Headgear	35
	Military Funeral	36
	Position of Honor	38
	Saluting	39

SECTION III.	Ceremonial & Social Protocol 42	
	Dining-In & Dining-Out	42
	Official Dinners & Receptions	46
	Presentation of Awards	53
	Promotion Ceremony	56
	Retirement Ceremony	59

SECTION IV.	Special Duty 64	
	Aide-de-Camp	64
	Boards	67
	Chief Professional Officer	68
	Escort Officer	69
	Honor Corps	73
	Junior Officer Advisory Group	76
	Liaison, Commissioned Corps	77
	Minority Officers Liaison Council	77
	Music Ensemble	79
	Professional Advisory Committee	80
	Protocol Officer	82
	Readiness Force	84
	Recruiter	87
	Surgeon General's Policy Advisory Council	88
SECTION V.	Communications 89	
	Business Cards	89
	Calls & Cards	91
	Conversation	93
	Correspondence	95
	Greetings & Introductions	100
	Presentations & Speaking	103
	Telecommunications	105
SECTION VI.	Meetings 108	
	The Chairperson	109
	The Participants	110
	Office Appointments	111
	Conventions	112
	Parliamentary Procedure	112

SECTION VII.	Table Protocol 115	
	Table Settings	115
	Table Manners	120
	Restaurant Dining	124
SECTION VIII.	U.S. Public Health Service 129	
	Mission	129
	Organization	130
	Office of the Surgeon General	132
	Agency Assignments	134
	Regular Corps	139
	PHS History	139
	PHS Flag	141
	PHS Seal	141
	PHS CC Seal	141
	PHS March	142
	PHS Coin	142
SECTION IX.	Uniformed Service Organizations ...143	
	Organization of All Military Services	143
	U.S. Air Force	145
	U.S. Army	146
	U.S. Coast Guard	147
	U.S. Marine Corps	148
	U.S. Navy	149
	National Oceanic & Atmospheric Administration Corps	150
	Abbreviations, Acronyms, & Glossary	151
	Selected References	155

Appendices	*157*
A. Planning a Dining-Out	*158*
B. Planning a Formal Reception	*160*
C. Planning for Awards/Promotion	
/Retirement Ceremony	*162*
D. Escort Officer	
Planning for a Distinguished Visitor	*164*
E. Deployment	
Suggested Items to Take	*167*
Notes	*170*
Index	*171*

FOREWORD

UNITED STATES SURGEON GENERAL

A U.S. PUBLIC HEALTH SERVICE COMMISSIONED OFFICER is characterized as someone having the requisite training and practical skills, considerable prowess as a public health professional, and a deep commitment to maintaining our most important national asset—the health of our people. We daily live the legacy, a proud heritage of service built over 200 years, dedicating ourselves to protecting, promoting, and advancing the health and safety of the Nation. Once confined to our national boundaries, the role of the Commissioned Corps has rapidly expanded to become global in nature—we now have the additional responsibility of responding to public health emergencies throughout the world.

As the only uniformed service comprised solely of health-related professionals, this ability presents us with new challenges. These challenges cannot be met alone, as we must achieve joint interoperability with other uniformed services and our civilian counterparts. Knowledge of the traditions, customs, protocols, and social etiquette that are so much a part of our sister services, and to some extent society in general, will enable us to better achieve seamless interactions. The importance of relating well with other persons is essential to ensuring cooperation and negotiating success. The capacity to do so also creates an enduring integrity and vitality within our Corps that will have significant impact on how we are viewed by others.

The *Public Health Service Officer's Guide* is an excellent reference in this area and provides an opportunity for officers to enhance their knowledge base. The *Guide* presents a comprehensive and organized review of uniformed service courtesies, customs, protocols, standards, and other pertinent information of benefit to all Commissioned Officers, regardless of their years of service. In concert with other resources, the *Guide* helps officers better understand these courtesies and customs and how best to implement them. Read the *Guide*—be confident and self-assured—our promise for the future begins with a well prepared Corps!

                              Richard H. Carmona, MD, MPH, FACS
                              VADM, USPHS
                              United States Surgeon General

My sincerest thanks to CAPT (ret.) James E. Knoben and CDR Alice Knoben for their dedication, commitment and devotion to the U.S. Public Health Service Commissioned Corps – they have created in the Public Health Service Officer's Guide a treasure for all of us.

Preface

THE UNITED STATES PUBLIC HEALTH SERVICE has a long and distinguished record of service to our Nation. Since its inception over two hundred years ago, PHS officers have confronted public health issues with vision, determination and compassion. Today, the Commissioned Corps has a breadth of medical expertise that places it in a unique leadership position to protect, promote, and advance public health.

The interdependent relationship of nations and world events in recent years have compelled the U.S. Public Health Service to transform itself in order to more effectively address medical challenges on a global scale. These new responsibilities require a greater level of preparedness and knowledge about providing health care in differing circumstances and in diverse cultures. In responding to emergent public health situations, nationally and internationally, the participation of PHS officers with other uniformed service personnel calls for seamless interoperability among the services. Such cooperative effort requires that PHS officers have a good understanding of military protocol to effectively carry out their duties. Further, for the PHS officer, a secure knowledge of military and social protocol may be essential in realizing successful health diplomacy.

The integration of military protocol with social consciousness is reflected by the adage "an officer and a gentleman." Uniformed service officers are judged by how they conduct themselves and relate to others, as well as their professional competence. All uniformed services of the United States provide officers with a knowledge of protocol and service tradition in order to enhance their officers' personal effectiveness, promote esprit de corps, and to effect a favorable working environment that impacts positively on overall productivity and corporate image of the uniformed service.

The heritage of the Public Health Service—its history, customs and traditions—is a foundation upon which PHS officers can continue the legacy of unparalleled accomplishment. The *Public Health Service Officer's Guide* provides officers with a concise source of information on uniformed service and PHS protocol, traditions, service standards, and etiquette that complements their heritage. It is hoped that, through use of this book, PHS officers will achieve a more rewarding professional life which will, in turn, serve to strengthen the U.S. Public Health Service Commissioned Corps as it advances forward in this new millennium.

ACKNOWLEDGMENTS

The writing of the *Public Health Service Officer's Guide* was a challenging, yet very worthwhile endeavor. The support of the Office of the Surgeon General, beginning with Surgeon General Richard H. Carmona and Deputy Surgeon General Kenneth Moritsugu, has been significantly important to the book's completion. The participation of OSG staff made this a collegial process that will benefit all PHS officers. In particular, we want to thank Rear Admiral Robert Williams, Chief of Staff, who led the review process within the OSG, and Lieutenant Patricio Garcia, Aide-de-Camp, who was an early participant. Other officers who provided thorough and thoughtful reviews of the manuscript included Rear Admiral John Babb, Captain Raymond Clark, Lieutenant Joshua Hardin, Captain Helena Mishoe, and Captain Gilbert Rose. Their comments were of enormous value in ensuring the accuracy and readability of the book.

It is noteworthy that many persons recognized the need for a PHS officer's guide and were quite supportive of the project. The collection of relevant information was a considerable effort and we are grateful to those who were a resource for essential details that enhanced the reliability of the book. We particularly want to recognize Dr. Alexandra Lord, PHS Historian, and CAPT Susanne Caviness for their contributions. Our thanks also to uniformed service officials who provided military guidance, especially Ms. Jo Ostendorf, Chief of Protocol at Whiteman Air Force Base.

Captain Jerry Farrell, USN (Ret.), Executive Director of the Commissioned Officers Association of the USPHS, Rear Admiral Jerrold Michael, USPHS (Ret.), President of the PHS Commissioned Officers Foundation for the Advancement of Public Health, and Trustees of the Foundation are to be commended for their role in providing the support needed to make this book available to PHS Commissioned Officers.

*This book is dedicated to the men and women
of the U.S. Public Health Service
who continue the heritage of public health leadership
in meeting the challenges of our Nation and the world.*

SECTION I.

UNIFORMED SERVICE BASICS

Uniformed service personnel transition between civilian and service life throughout their career. The nature of being a commissioned officer, however, requires a person to learn about the personal qualities and identifying features that differentiate an officer from a civilian. This section covers some of the basics, including the importance of protocol and tradition; what is expected of a commissioned officer; uniformed service ranks and insignia; and, service uniforms.

> PROTOCOL AND TRADITION
> USPHS AND OFFICERSHIP
> LEADERSHIP
> PERSONNEL, RANKS AND INSIGNIA
> UNIFORM AND DEVICE STANDARDS

Protocol and Tradition

In most societies and institutions, there are prescribed behavioral norms and ceremonies to mark life events. These observances often derive from customs, protocol and tradition that develop over hundreds of years. Their importance transcends the mere collective practice of a form of conduct or activity. Rather, when morally-based, such practice weaves a social fabric through the society that joins people together in greater harmony, and further provides a bond with past and future generations.

Uniformed services place great emphasis on the observance of protocol and tradition. Protocol includes the military courtesies and customs that show respect for others and foster good human relationships. Traditions represent the accumulated experiences of the uniformed services and its service members that are passed forward.

The heritage of each service includes the protocol, customs and traditions that impart esprit de corps and individual pride in being a member of that particular uniformed service. Service heritage has many facets, among which are experiences relating to the institution itself or the environment in which it operates (e.g., nautical customs of the U.S. Navy), the historical record of the institution in carrying out its mission, and to individual or group feats of noteworthy accomplishment or heroism. This heritage is at once a foundation and an inspiration for present-day uniformed service members to meet challenges with the courage and resolve shown by their forebears.

As with other uniformed services, the heritage of the U.S. Public Health Service (USPHS or PHS) is profound in terms of its impact on the well-being of our fellow citizens and people around the world. PHS officers are beneficiaries of this record of public health leadership and continue that tradition today.

There are many customs and traditions shared by all uniformed services. These relate to the protocol, ceremonies, social and service standards that personnel learn upon joining a uniformed service. These customs may be modified to reflect the distinctive characteristics of each service and changed periodically in response to new trends, yet all are meant to enrich a person's professional career and social interactions within and outside the uniformed service. The value of embracing custom and tradition in uniformed service life has stood the test of time. PHS commissioned officers who understand the significance of doing so will benefit greatly.

USPHS and Officership

The U.S. Public Health Service is one of seven uniformed services of the United States of America that protect the welfare of our Nation, with each service contributing in its own way to realize that mission.

The USPHS is distinct due to its principal mission of protecting and promoting public health. PHS officers distinguish themselves by the array of healthcare responsibilities they hold—they are leaders in healthcare delivery, public health management, biomedical research, disease control, health protection, and health education on a global scale. Though the roles may differ, the commonality of purpose is a unifying force.

PHS officers work in clinical, administrative, regulatory and scientific positions. As a commissioned officer with essential public health responsibilities, the U.S. Public Health Service is an organization that is collegial and professional, and at the same time supportive of an officer Corps. By accepting a commission, PHS officers enter a service life with similar constraints, rights and privileges of officers in other uniformed services. In addition, certain personal qualities are important in a commissioned officer. The following is a discussion of officership—the qualities expected of a commissioned officer.

Officership

There is no universal definition of officership. Officership can be described as the essence of being an officer—an expectation that officers use professional judgment, possess moral fiber and values, and understand the relationship of the Corps and its role in service to society. A commonly held definition of officership among uniformed services is that it is a blend of leadership, management, and professionalism. For the PHS, characteristics of officership include the following:

- Competence—both as technical expert and a professional officer
- Knowledge, skills, and expertise as a public health professional
- Core values (excellence, integrity, loyalty, responsibility)
- Commitment to a common mission
- Ability as a leader and manager

All five aspects are important. Some indicators of officership that express the professionalism of being a USPHS commissioned officer include actions that demonstrate one's capabilities as a public health professional; competence in your assigned billet; serving on deployments; mentoring; teaching; participation on Corps related committees and task groups; and publications.

Officership also requires that commissioned officers always be aware of their attitudes and actions, and their interactive relationships with colleagues.

Attitude and Actions. Commissioned officers have a responsibility to conduct themselves appropriately. Appropriate conduct relates to one's attitude and actions—an officer's mind-set in performing his/her duties and how the officer relates to other uniformed service personnel, government officials and the public. By electing to become a member of a uniformed service, PHS officers accept that they are part of a hierarchical structure with certain prescribed features. They agree to conform to the conventions of uniformed service protocol and observe military behavior and courtesies that would be appropriate, such as the proper exchange of salutes between uniformed personnel. When in uniform, officers are expected to practice discipline in managing their personal feelings in order to place service before self. The "military way" is to accomplish a mission, whether a routine assignment in the office or an order given on the battle field. Officers complete their mission by performance of duty with excellence, bottom line.

Teamwork. The nature of a uniformed service is such that it is operationally best and most successful when a teamwork approach is used. Therefore, service personnel must be respectful of one another, cooperate with others and work together for the common good, keeping foremost in mind the overall mission. With mission in mind, good officers will stand ready to help other officers succeed in their respective duty roles.

Personal ambition and competition are appropriate when an officer or group of officers is striving for excellence—the officer and service can benefit from such effort. However, personal ambition has no place in a uniformed service if it is unethical or injurious to others. Officers must make a conscious effort to think how their actions affect others and adjust their actions and motivations, accordingly.

Leadership

The characteristics of officership include several qualities, but chief among these is leadership. Effective leadership is key to ensuring that personnel are fulfilled in their roles, that teamwork flourishes, and a quality outcome is attained. Commissioned officers are called upon to be leaders in every way. PHS officers need to understand the importance of good leadership ability and seek leadership training early in their career. There are many definitions of leadership. Generally stated:

> *Leadership is the ability to influence others by strength of character and personal vision to achieve common goals.*

Military officers are taught to be leaders. The reason is evident—the military exists to defend and protect our Nation, and that entails fighting wars. When going into battle, losing is not an option and, thus, military leaders courageously lead soldiers into battle for the common good. Although not all military personnel serve in combat, all military people take their responsibilities seriously, sharing a unity of purpose that places great emphasis on duty, honor, and Country.

PHS officers, though not an armed force, share a common purpose with other uniformed services in supporting the welfare of our Nation. In fulfilling their responsibilities, PHS officers are leaders by carrying out their duties with integrity, by keeping their focus on service before self, and by taking initiative to make the world a better place.

Leadership Theories
There are various leadership theories. For example, the *trait* theory defines a leadership profile in terms of distinguishing personal traits, such as intelligence, integrity, courage, etc. The *behavioral* theory relies on observations of leadership behavior and leadership styles, such as directive/production-centered or participative/people-centered. The *situational* leadership theory notes that effective leadership is dependent upon, and must adapt to the surrounding environment and state of events. *Transformational* leadership refers to the leader as a charismatic visionary who inspires and motivates others for change. Each of these theories contribute to an individual's leadership approach, and all provide insight into useful attribute and skill development.

Attributes, Skills, and Core Competencies
In a study by the Army War College, the following attributes of a leader were listed (in order of importance):
- Keeps cool under pressure
- Clearly explains missions, standards, and priorities
- Sees the big picture, providing context and perspective
- Makes tough, sound decisions on time
- Adapts quickly to new situations; can handle bad news
- Gives useful feedback
- Sets a high ethical tone
- Is positive, encouraging, and realistically optimistic

Most leadership training focuses on the development of skills and abilities, which are combined with an awareness of personal attributes, experiences, and environmental influences. The Federal Office of Personnel Management's Senior Executive Service has identified five Executive Core Qualifications to describe the critical leadership skills needed to succeed, which are built upon core competencies. The following excerpts are illustrative:
- Leading change
  The ability to implement an organizational vision which integrates program goals and priorities, balances change with continuity (continually improves customer service and program performance), and encourages creative thinking.
  Competencies: creativity, resilience, service motivation, strategic thinking.
- Leading people
  The ability to implement strategies that maximize employee potential and foster high ethical standards in meeting the organization's vision, mission, and goals.
  Competencies: honesty, integrity, team building, leverage (value) diversity.
- Results driven
  The ability to stress accountability and continuous improvement, make timely and effective decisions, and to produce results through strategic planning.
  Competencies: accountability, decisive, problem solving, technical credibility.
- Business acumen
  The ability to acquire and administer human, financial, material and information resources in a manner that instills public trust and accomplishes the mission.
  Competencies: financial-, human resources-, and technology management.
- Building coalitions/communication
  The ability to express facts and ideas in a convincing manner, negotiate with individuals/groups internally and externally, develop a professional network with other organizations, and identify factors that impact the work of the organization.
  Competencies: interpersonal skills, communication abilities, partnering.

To be an effective leader, one must begin to develop core competencies. These broadly include knowledge, problem-solving skills, and social judgment skills. Throughout one's career in the Public Health Service, there is a need for officers to continually develop their core competencies. Depending on where you are within your career, different competencies may be emphasized more than others, and perhaps at different levels of significance. A Lieutenant may need more technical competency, whereas a Captain would require more personnel relationship and conceptual competencies. Lifelong learning and enhancement of core competencies is imperative to success in the Commissioned Corps, as well as any aspect of business or personal life. In addition to learning leadership principles and skill sets, practical application of that knowledge is required. We are only leaders if others perceive us to be. Officers need to show leadership through actions that exemplify a good leader. For example, do officers take initiative to lead a group effort, seek solutions to challenging situations, or provide strategic vision for their program?

Leadership Principles and Qualities
Much is written about principles and qualities that typify a good leader—the following is a synopsis of some of those qualities.
Self-Knowledge. First, know yourself. This is a fundamental truth, for unless a person first learns about himself, it will be difficult to progress. Honestly evaluate your strengths and deficiencies, moral and ethical stances, likes and dislikes, and life goals. The objective is to know your baseline and the areas you want to improve upon. Take initiative to improve yourself through reading, listening, observing, taking training, and seeking others' opinions. Having a good mentor or role model is particularly important in this endeavor.
Integrity. Integrity is a hallmark of the good officer. What you stand for, and whether you are willing to stand up for what is right will affect your decisions throughout your career. Your performance of duties and professional relations with others must be consistently ethical, since other officers will determine their level of trust in you on the basis of your honesty and character. Senior officers set the tone of an organization—they must act honorably for the organization to flourish. Transparency of process and accountability are essential features of corporate integrity. Senior officers are cognizant of the importance of acting responsibly and taking the high road when they make official decisions. They must be vigilant to promote equity towards subordinates; to do otherwise will undermine their authority and weaken esprit de corps within the officer Corps.
Competency. Every officer should be proficient in his/her chosen profession and life's work. Throughout his career, there are opportunities for an officer to broaden his professional knowledge and experience, oftentimes in areas that might not directly relate to the entry profession. Seek out these opportunities and learn about the PHS, past and present, in order to attain a solid grounding and true sense of purpose in mission fulfillment.
Respect for Others. Sensitivity to the rights, beliefs and needs of others is a leadership trait. This applies both to one's fellow officers and to those we serve. Practice being a good listener, because it is essential to be well informed in order to be most effective. Communicate your thoughts clearly and transparently. Ensure that others understand the importance of their role in a mission and recognize the contribution of their efforts in its accomplishment.

Taking Responsibility. Commitment to accomplishing the PHS mission entails taking responsibility in several ways. All officers should become involved in support activities that strengthen the PHS. The PHS will only be effective if its officers take personal responsibility for the ongoing improvement of PHS programs and systems. Officers show commitment by taking ownership of identified problems and seeing them through to complete resolution. Officers need to be decisive in carrying out their duties, and accountable for their decisions and actions. And, officers must assume responsibility for their behavior within and outside the uniformed service. These are all important indicators of an increased level of maturity.

PHS officers will find that those who serve the public health mission with excellence and with respect for others derive enjoyment and gratification in their work. Further, those who make the effort to maintain a positive attitude in spite of setbacks, move forward with fortitude, and work to improve the Commissioned Corps will receive great personal satisfaction and self-respect.

Personnel, Ranks and Insignia

There are seven uniformed services of the United States: the Public Health Service, Air Force, Army, Coast Guard, Marine Corps, National Oceanic and Atmospheric Administration, and Navy. Within the seven uniformed services are three categories of military personnel: commissioned officers, warrant officers, and enlisted personnel.

Commissioned Officers
Commissioned officers have a four-year bachelor's degree, and may need a master's degree to be promoted. Officers are commissioned through programs such as the military service academies (Air Force Academy at Colorado Springs, U.S. Military Academy at West Point, Coast Guard Academy at New London, Naval Academy at Annapolis), Reserve Officer Training Corps, Officer Candidate School, or Officer Training School (Air Force).
  There are ten commissioned officer grades:
  Pay Grades O-1 to O-3
    Junior grade officers—Coast Guard, Navy, NOAA, PHS
    Company grade officers—Air Force, Army, Marine Corps
  Pay Grades O-4 to O-6
    Senior grade officers—Coast Guard, Navy, NOAA, PHS
    Field grade officers—Air Force, Army, Marine Corps
  Pay Grades O-7 to O-10
    Flag officers—Coast Guard, Navy, NOAA, PHS
    General/flag officers—Air Force, Army, Marine Corps

Military officers may be generally classified as line and non-line officers. Unrestricted line officers are trained combat specialists, whereas non-line officers are considered staff officers with specialty training (e.g., Supply Corps).

Warrant Officers
Warrant officers may receive direct warrant commissions or be advanced from the enlisted ranks based on training and experience. Though not required, many warrant officers have college degrees. There are five warrant officer grades. These officers hold warrants and are experts and specialists in certain capabilities or technologies, and serve as "middle managers" within the military structure. Upon promotion to chief warrant officer 2, they become commissioned warrant officers. There are no warrant officers in the Air Force.

Enlisted Personnel
Enlisted personnel are required to have a high school diploma to join the military services. Following basic training, enlisted personnel are provided specialized training to perform the front-line jobs. There are nine enlisted pay grades, E-1 through E-9. Those in pay grades E-1 through E-3 are usually in training status (basic, specialized, advanced) or on their first assignment. The term used to identify a military person's specialty is *Air Force specialty* (Air Force), *military occupational specialty* (Army and Marine Corps), or *rating* (Navy). In the Navy, a rating badge on the uniform combines a unique rating insignia with the pay grade insignia (symbol above the stripes/chevrons).

Upon reaching the E-4/E-5 through E-9 grades, enlisted personnel achieve a leadership status known as **noncommissioned officer** (NCO) status. NCO status begins at the grade E-4/5 in the Army (corporal/sergeant), E-5 in the Air Force (staff sergeant), and E-4 in the Marine Corps (corporal). The equivalent to NCO in the Navy and Coast Guard is the petty officer, which begins at the grade E-4 (petty officer third class). At the E-8 and E-9 levels, there may be two positions at the same pay grade depending on the job performed. The top E-9 levels are reserved for the senior enlisted person of each uniformed service, each of whom is the spokesperson of their respective enlisted force.

Ranks and Insignia
The badges of rank have evolved over thousands of years of military history. Beginning with the Revolutionary War, American ranks and insignia were designed as adaptations of the British tradition. The specific ranks and insignia used among the uniformed services vary. Generally, the U.S. Coast Guard, Navy, NOAA, and Public Health Service have the same ranks and insignia for commissioned personnel and enlisted (Coast Guard and Navy) personnel. Among the U.S. Air Force, Army, and Marine Corps, ranks and insignia are the same for commissioned personnel, but differ for enlisted personnel. Each service has a unique service crest. *(See the charts, Rank Insignia, pages 9-14.)*

UNIFORMED SERVICE BASICS

ENLISTED RANK INSIGNIA

	ARMY	NAVY, COAST GRD	MARINE CORPS	AIR FORCE
E1	Private	Seaman Recruit (SR)	Private	Airman Basic
E2	Private E-2 (PV2)	Seaman Apprentice (SA)	Private First Class (PFC)	Airman (Amn)
E3	Private First Class (PFC)	Seaman (SN)	Lance Corporal (LCpl)	Airman First Class (A1C)
E4	Corporal (CPL) Specialist (SPC)	Petty Officer Third Class (PO3)	Corporal (Cpl)	Senior Airman (SrA)
E5	Sergeant (SGT)	Petty Officer Second Class (PO2)	Sergeant (Sgt)	Staff Sergeant (SSgt)
E6	Staff Sergeant (SSG)	Petty Officer First Class (PO1)	Staff Sergeant (SSgt)	Technical Sergeant (TSgt)

ENLISTED RANK INSIGNIA *(Continued)*

	ARMY		NAVY, COAST GRD		MARINE CORPS			AIR FORCE
E7	Sergeant First Class (SFC)		Chief Petty Officer (CPO)		Gunnery Sergeant (GySgt)		Master Sergeant (MSgt)	First Sergeant
E8	Master Sergeant (MSG)	First Sergeant (1SG)	Senior Chief Petty Officer (SCPO)		Master Sergeant (MSgt)	First Sergeant	Senior Master Sergeant (SMSgt)	First Sergeant
E9	Sergeant Major (SGM)	Command Sergeant Major (CSM)	Master Chief Petty Officer (MCPO)	Fleet/Command Master Chief Petty Officer	Sergeant Major (SgtMaj)	Master Gunnery Sergeant (MGySgt)	Chief Master Sergeant (CMSgt)	First Sergeant	Command Chief Master Sergeant (CCM)
E9	Sergeant Major of the Army (SMA)		Master Chief Petty Officer of the Navy (MCPON) and Coast Guard (MCPOCG)		Sergeant Major of the Marine Corps (SgtMajMC)			Chief Master Sergeant of the Air Force (CMSAF)

UNIFORMED SERVICE BASICS **11**

WARRANT OFFICER RANK INSIGNIA

	ARMY	NAVY, COAST GRD	MARINE CORPS	AIR FORCE
W1	Warrant Officer 1 WO1	USN Warrant Officer 1 — WO1	Warrant Officer 1 WO	NO WARRANT
W2	Chief Warrant Officer 2 CW2	USN Chief Warrant Officer 2 — CWO2 / USCG	Chief Warrant Officer 2 CWO2	NO WARRANT
W3	Chief Warrant Officer 3 CW3	USN Chief Warrant Officer 3 — CWO3 / USCG	Chief Warrant Officer 3 CWO3	NO WARRANT
W4	Chief Warrant Officer 4 CW4	USN Chief Warrant Officer 4 — CWO4 / USCG	Chief Warrant Officer 4 CWO4	NO WARRANT
W5	Chief Warrant Officer CW5	USN Chief Warrant Officer CWO5	Chief Warrant Officer 5 CWO5	NO WARRANT

12 PHS Officer's Guide

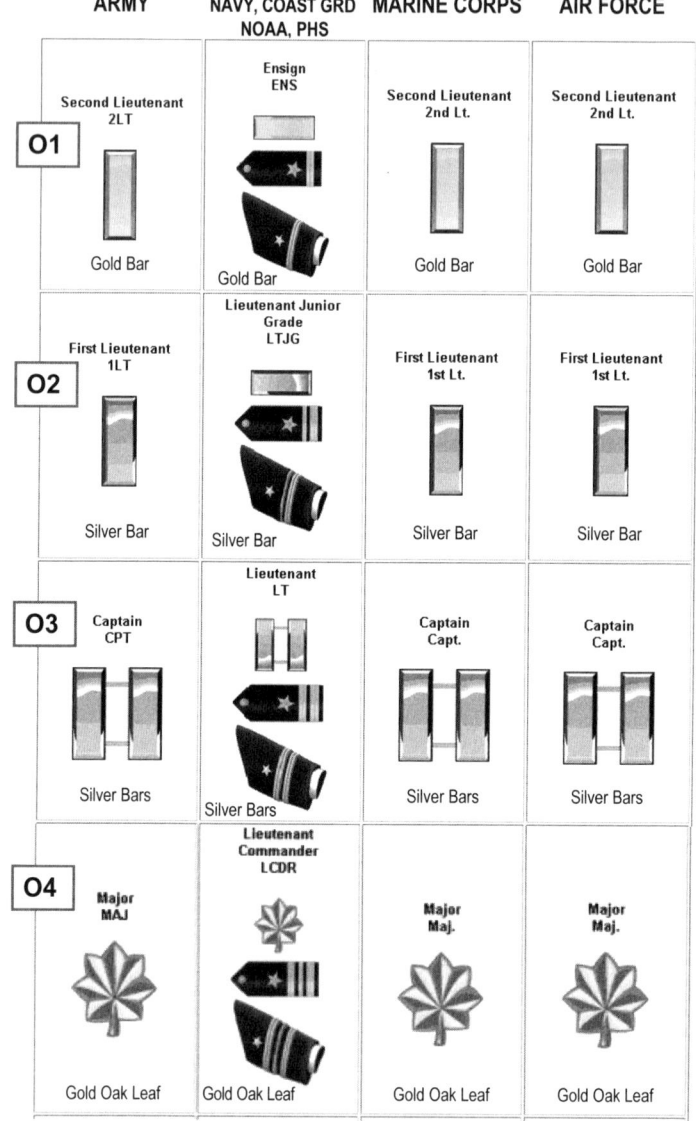

UNIFORMED SERVICE BASICS 13

COMMISSIONED OFFICER RANK INSIGNIA *(Continued)*

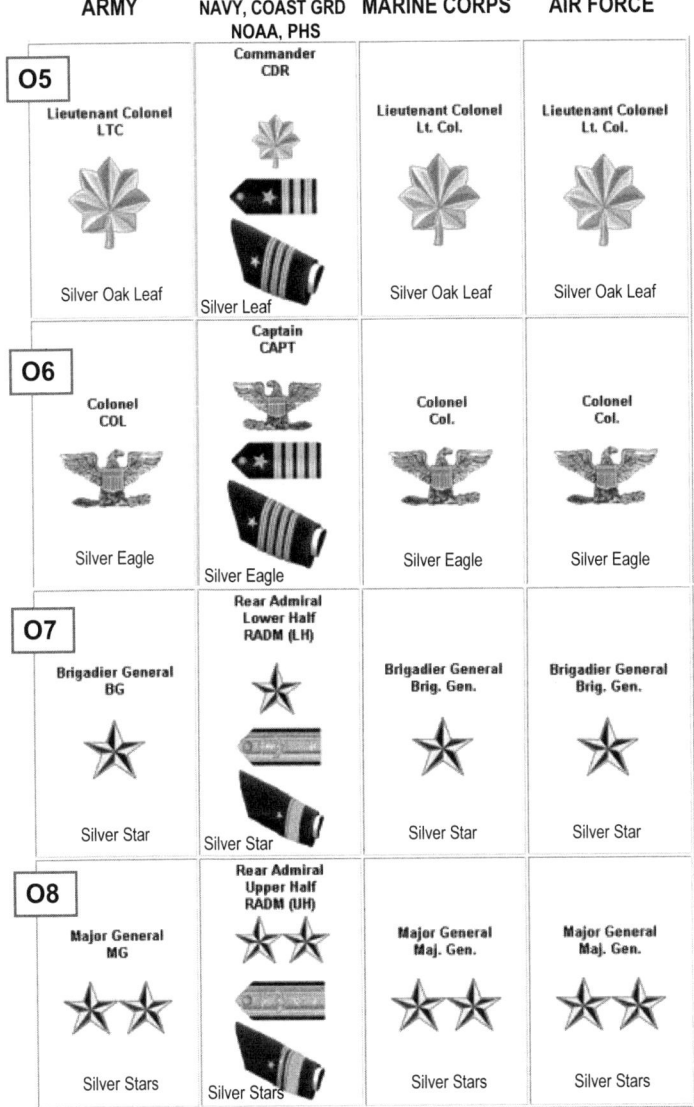

COMMISSIONED OFFICER RANK INSIGNIA *(Continued)*

	ARMY	NAVY, COAST GRD NOAA, PHS	MARINE CORPS	AIR FORCE
O9	Lieutenant General LTG — Silver Stars	Vice Admiral VADM — Silver Stars	Lieutenant General Lt. Gen. — Silver Stars	Lieutenant General Lt. Gen. — Silver Stars
O10	General GEN Army Chief of Staff — Silver Stars	Admiral ADM Chief of Naval Operations and Commandant of the Coast Guard — Silver Stars	General Gen. Commandant of the Marine Corps — Silver Stars	General Gen. Air Force Chief of Staff — Silver Stars
	General of the Army (Reserved for wartime only) — Silver Stars	Fleet Admiral (Reserved for wartime only) — Silver Stars	(None)	General of the Air Force (Reserved for wartime only) — Silver Stars

Source: U.S. Department of Defense Defenselink Website.

Uniform and Device Standards

U.S. Public Health Service uniforms are generally comprised of the same articles of clothing used by the U.S. Navy, with the exception of some optional and special-purpose uniforms. PHS uniforms are made distinctive by the wearing of unique PHS insignia, including the Corps device, cap chin strap, cap device, shoulder boards, insignia, name tag, and buttons.

The uniform is a key element in presenting a proper uniformed service image, coupled with a well groomed personal appearance. Officers serve as role models and are therefore expected to maintain the highest standards when wearing the uniform. Uniformed service personnel typically wear the uniform daily while on duty, and officers need to be cognizant of the importance of proper grooming and compliance with uniform standards.

The following information highlights those features of personal grooming and uniform standards about which officers should be knowledgeable. For more detailed information, refer to official PHS Personnel Instructions and Directives.

Personal Appearance and Grooming
Hair. *Men's hair* must be clean and neatly trimmed. Hair shall be no longer than 4 inches and may not touch the ears and shirt collar on the back, nor extend below the eyebrows. The hair should not show under the front edge of headgear nor interfere with the proper wearing of any headgear. The bulk of hair may not exceed approximately 2 inches. Sideburns must not extend below a point level with the middle of the ear, shall be of even width (not flared) and end on a horizontal line. Hair coloring and hairpieces shall be natural in appearance. Mustaches must not cover the lip line of the upper lip and, absent a beard, may not extend outward (and not downward) more than ¼ inch beyond the corners of the mouth. Unlike the armed forces, the PHS does allow beards, but only if they are full or partial (not patches), neatly trimmed and the bulk does not exceed ½ inch in length.

Women's hair must be clean, neatly styled, and present a balanced and generally conservative appearance. Hair coloring and hairpieces or wigs shall be natural in appearance. The hair on all sides may touch, but not fall below a horizontal line level with the lower edge of the back of the shirt collar. Hair should not show below the front brim of headgear, nor should the hairstyle interfere with the proper wearing of any headgear. Long hair which would otherwise fall below the edge of the collar shall be neatly fastened, pinned or secured to the head with plain bobby pins, small barrettes/combs/clips similar to hair color. Alligator clips, fabric elastic bands (scrunchies) and hair ornaments are not authorized. Hair bulk may not exceed approximately 2 inches.

Body Alterations. No tattoos/body art are permitted on the head, face, neck or scalp. Tattoos are deemed unacceptable if visually offensive due to large size, obscene or prejudicial content. Intentional body mutilation, (e.g., piercing, branding, scarring) on the head, face, neck or scalp are prohibited. Women may pierce their earlobes for wearing earrings. Women may wear nail polish, but it must be a single conservative color that complements the skin tone.

Personal Articles, Eyeglasses, Jewelry, Watches. When in uniform, personal articles such as pens, combs and handkerchiefs shall be kept in pockets or otherwise not be visible upon the uniform. Eyeglasses, including sunglasses, must be conservative in design. Jewelry should be conservative and kept to a minimum. Only one ring per hand is authorized, plus a wedding/engagement ring. Earrings are not authorized for men. Women may wear 4 mm-6 mm ball earrings, plain with shiny or brushed matte finish, one gold earring per ear with all uniforms. Small single pearl earrings are authorized with Dinner Dress and Formal uniforms. Only one necklace may be worn and it shall not be visible. One conservative wristwatch and one bracelet may be worn on the same or different arms; ankle bracelets are not authorized. Jewelry shall not present a safety hazard.

Bags and Communication Devices

Bags (e.g., briefcase, gym bag, backpack, laptop bag, lunch bag, suitcase, garment bag) are carried in the left hand. However, backpacks, gym, laptop and garment bags may be worn with the strap over the left shoulder of BDUs, service and working uniforms (e.g., khaki uniforms), and backpacks may be worn over both shoulders of working uniforms; all such bags may be worn when riding a bicycle or motorcycle. All bags must conceal their contents and be either black or navy blue, with no ornamentation except the PHS logo in yellow or the bag manufacturer's logo (if small). All bags shall be hand carried when in "dress" uniform.

Communication devices (e.g., cellular phone, pager, personal digital assistant) may be worn on the belt of service and working uniforms, on either side of the body and behind the elbow, such that they are not visible from the front. For service dress and more formal uniforms, these devices are to be worn so as not to be visible, nor affect the appearance of the uniform (i.e., bulging or protruding on the front, side or rear).

Headgear

There are five principal types of headgear prescribed for PHS officers.

The *combination* or *service cap* is the standard officer's cap with black visor and distinctive device and ornamentation. The cap is covered in white or khaki material, as appropriate. The combination cap is worn squarely on the head, with the bottom edge parallel to and approximately ½ inch above the eyebrows.

The *garrison cap* is Navy blue with gold piping or khaki material. The garrison cap is worn squarely on the head, with fore and aft crease centered vertically between the eyebrows, with the lowest point of the cap approximately ½ inch above the eyebrows.

The *beret,* authorized for women, is black. The beret is worn toward the front of the head, approximately ¾ inch from the forehead hairline, and tilted slightly to the right.

The command *ball cap* is black, with "U.S. PUBLIC HEALTH SERVICE" embroidered in golden yellow across the top front panel. The cap is worn squarely on the head, with the bottom edge parallel to the ground and approximately ½ inch above the top of the ears.

The *utility cap* is Woodland Green camouflage pattern, Navy-style with six sides and firm bill. The utility cap is worn squarely on the head.

Name Tag
The PHS name tag is a required component of the service uniforms and may be worn with working uniforms; it is not worn with ceremonial, formal, or dinner dress uniforms. The name tag is positioned on the right side of the uniform coat, with the lower edge of the tag centered ¼ inch above the same relative position as the left breast pocket.

Uniform Considerations
Uniforms should be procured only after the officer is completely familiar with prescribed design and specifications. Note that uniform components which are described as *blue* color refer to the Navy blue authorized material that is black in appearance. Each uniform needs to be tailored to fit properly, maintained in good condition and replaced whenever necessary. Keep uniforms clean and pressed (military creases recommended), and shoes shined and in good repair. Fabric badges, insignia and ribbons need to be kept clean and, if frayed, replaced. Metallic devices such as the belt buckle should be clean and bright, and replaced if scratched. The gig line, which includes the shirt placket, belt buckle and trouser fly, are properly kept in vertical alignment.

Uniform Classifications
PHS uniforms can be placed into five categories:

<u>General Purpose Service Uniforms</u>
    Service Dress Blue
    Service Dress Blue Sweater
    Service Dress White
    Service Blue (Salt & Pepper)
    Service Khaki
    Summer White
    Winter Blue

<u>Working Uniforms</u>
    Working Khaki
    Indoor Duty White
    Winter Working Blue

Special Situation Uniforms
    Battle Dress
    Maternity

Ceremonial Uniforms
    Full Dress Blue
    Full Dress White

Formal and Dinner Dress Uniforms
    Formal Dress
    Dinner Dress Blue Jacket
    Dinner Dress White Jacket
    Dinner Dress Blue
    Dinner Dress White
    Tropical Dinner Dress Blue

The principal features of these uniforms are provided in the tables "Basic Uniform Components, Male/Female" on pages 25-28.

Uniform Policy
Uniform of the Day. PHS officers may wear only those uniforms that are prescribed by the Local Uniform Authority. Additionally, Service Dress Blue is always acceptable in a normal office setting. Wearing of the PHS uniform is required while on official duty, in accordance with the directives of competent PHS or agency authority.
Other Uniformed Service. PHS officers assigned to the U.S. Coast Guard wear the uniform prescribed for wear by Coast Guard officers, but with PHS insignia. PHS officers assigned to a uniformed service other than the Coast Guard for extended active duty shall, if required under the provisions of the assignment agreement, wear the uniform prescribed for that service. If the agreement does not specify that the officer is to wear the uniform of the service to which assigned, nor does it prohibit the wearing of the PHS uniform, the PHS officer shall wear the PHS uniform that corresponds to the type of uniform prescribed for wear by officers of the other service.
Retired Officers. Retired and Reserve Corps officers not on active duty may wear the prescribed PHS uniform of the rank held on the retired or inactive list on occasions of ceremony and at gatherings of organizations comprised primarily of uniformed service members. Wearing of BDUs during emergency responses or exercises thereof when part of a team with active duty officers may be allowed, provided a civilian patch is worn. Wearing of the uniform for other occasions or purposes is prohibited.
Travel. For official domestic travel, a PHS officer may wear the uniform of the day prescribed for the area to which the officer is proceeding.

When travel is by non-military conveyance within the United States, a PHS officer may wear Service Dress Blue, the uniform specified in orders, or appropriate civilian attire.

For official and unofficial travel by military-owned or -controlled conveyance, a PHS officer is authorized to wear civilian clothing. However, PHS officers are also authorized and encouraged to wear the PHS uniform for military travel. The officer shall wear the uniform when travelers belonging to the uniformed service that is providing the conveyance are required to travel in uniform. If military officials advise that foreign entry requirements prohibit wearing the uniform, or that the officer will be passing through high-risk areas relating to terrorist activities, or political or social unrest, the uniform shall not be worn.

For international travel, in accordance with international agreements, PHS officers are generally not permitted to wear the uniform outside the United States unless the Surgeon General gives authorization or the officer is assigned to another uniformed service whose regulations permit wearing the uniform.

Insignia
Cap. The *combination cap* is worn with the standard size cap device, centered on the front of the hat band, with ornamentation that varies with grade: LCDR and below, no ornamentation; CAPT and CDR, the male officer's visor is embroidered with gold oak leaves and acorns, and the female officer's hat band is embroidered with one row of gold oak leaves and acorns; flag officer, the male officer's visor is fully embroidered with gold oak leaves and acorns, and the female officer's hat band is embroidered with two rows of gold oak leaves and acorns.

The *garrison cap* is worn with a miniature metal grade insignia on the right and a miniature PHS cap device on the left. The devices are centered 1¼ inches from the front center line crease and 1¼ inches from the lower edge of the cap. Captain's grade officers wear the right eagle (i.e., eagle's head points toward the center line).

The *beret* is worn with a miniature PHS cap device positioned so as to be aligned over the left eye; no grade insignia are worn on the beret.

Collar. Grade insignia, though similar among the uniformed services, are not always placed on the collar. Placement is the same for PHS and Naval officers. Miniature metal grade insignia are worn on the right collar points of blue and khaki shirts.

For long sleeve shirts, the center of the grade insignia is 1 inch from the front and upper edges of the collar. Bar- and leaf-shaped (tip point up) insignia are vertically aligned and parallel with the front edge of the collar; the right eagle is vertically aligned and parallel with the front edge of the collar; and for flag officers, the first star is positioned 1 inch from the front and upper edges of the collar, with any remaining stars extending back and parallel with the upper collar edge, with one ray of each star pointing up.

For open collar short sleeve shirts, the center of the grade insignia is 1 inch from the front and lower edges of the collar. The vertical axis of the insignia bisects the angle of the collar point.

A miniature metal Corps device is worn on the left collar, centered 1 inch from the appropriate collar edges, as described above, with the staff of the caduceus vertically aligned and the anchor points toward the front.

Shoulder. Hard and soft shoulder boards consist of a Corps device and grade indication, and the hard shoulder boards also have a PHS gilt button. Each shoulder board is positioned with the squared end at the shoulder seam and the Corps device towards the neck. The anchors of the Corps device are positioned such that each anchor points forward (hence the saying, "don't drag your anchors") when the boards are worn on the correct shoulder.

Awards and Badges

Awards and decorations that are awarded to service members give public recognition to exceptional accomplishments and performance of duties. These awards are manifested by medals and ribbons worn on an officer's uniform. The placement and order of precedence is prescribed for all awards, including those received by PHS officers while serving in other uniformed services. In all cases of relative priority, PHS awards take precedence over other uniformed service awards.

Order of Precedence. PHS officers wear uniformed service awards and decorations in the following order of precedence:
    PHS Honor Awards and Uniformed Services Decorations
    Unit Awards
    Non-Uniformed Service Decorations
    PHS Service and Campaign Awards
    Military Campaign, Service and Training Awards
    Foreign Decorations and Non-U.S. Service Awards
    Foreign Unit Awards
    Non-U.S. Service Awards
    PHS Regular Corps Ribbon
    Military Society and Organizational Awards

PHS Honor Awards and Uniformed Service Decorations
The order of precedence is as follows.
    Medal of Honor (Army, Navy, Air Force)
    Army Distinguished Service Cross
    Navy Cross
    Air Force Cross
    Defense Distinguished Service Medal
    Distinguished Service Medal/Valor (PHS)
    Distinguished Service Medal (PHS)
    Distinguished Service Medal (Other Services)
    Silver Star Medal
    Dept. of Transportation (DOT) Secretary's
      Award for Outstanding Achievement

DOT Gold Medal (Coast Guard)
Commerce Gold Medal (NOAA)
Defense Superior Service Medal
Meritorious Service Medal/Valor (PHS)
Meritorious Service Medal (PHS)
Surgeon General's Medallion (PHS)
Commerce Silver Medal (NOAA)
Surgeon General's Exemplary Service Medal (PHS)
Legion of Merit
Distinguished Flying Cross
Soldier's Medal (Army)
Navy & Marine Corps Medal
Airman's Medal (Air Force)
Coast Guard Medal
Gold Lifesaving Medal (Coast Guard)
Bronze Star Medal
Purple Heart
Defense Meritorious Service Medal
Outstanding Service Medal/Valor (PHS)
Outstanding Service Medal
Meritorious Service Medal (Other Services)
Commerce Bronze Medal (NOAA)
Air Medal
NOAA Administrator's Award
Silver Lifesaving Medal (Coast Guard)
DOT Secretary's Award for Meritorious Achievement
DOT Silver Medal (Coast Guard)
Aerial Achievement Medal
Joint Service Commendation Medal
Commendation Medal (PHS)
Commendation Medal (Other Services)
DOT Award for Superior Achievement
DOT Bronze Medal (Coast Guard)
Joint Service Achievement Medal
Achievement Medal (PHS)
Achievement Medal (Other Services)
Commerce Special Achievement Medal (NOAA)
PHS Citation
Commandant's Letter of Commendation Ribbon Bar
NOAA Corps Director's Award
Combat Action Ribbon (Navy, Coast Guard)

Unit Awards

The order of precedence is as follows.

Presidential Unit Citation (All Services)
Joint Meritorious Unit Award
Outstanding Unit Citation (PHS)
Valorous Unit Award (Army)
Air Force Outstanding Unit Award
DOT Outstanding Unit Award (Coast Guard)
Unit Commendation (PHS)

Unit Commendation Ribbon (All Services)
Meritorious Unit Commendation (All Services)
Army Superior Unit Award
Coast Guard Meritorious Team Commendation
Navy "E" Ribbon
Coast Guard "E" Ribbon
Air Force Organizational Excellence Award
Bicentennial Unit Commendation (PHS)
Coast Guard Bicentennial Unit Commendation

Non-Uniformed Service Decorations
The order of precedence conforms to the acceptance date.
Presidential Medal of Freedom
Medal for Merit
President's Distinguished Federal Civilian Service Medal
Bureau of Prisons (BOP) Distinguished Service Medal
Environmental Protection Agency (EPA) Gold Medal
BOP Meritorious Service Medal
EPA Silver Medal
BOP Commendation Medal
EPA Bronze Medal
EPA Distinguished Career Award

PHS Service and Campaign Awards
The order of precedence conforms to the acceptance date.
Crisis Response Service Award
Foreign Duty Award
Global Response Service Award
Hazardous Duty Award
Isolated/Hardship Award
National Emergency Preparedness Award
Special Assignment Award
Smallpox Eradication Campaign Ribbon

Military Campaign, Service, and Training Awards
Only PHS Awards are listed. See the Commissioned Corps Personnel Manual [CCPM] for other Uniformed Service awards.
Regular Corps Ribbon
Commissioned Corps Training Ribbon

Foreign Decorations and Non-U.S. Service Awards
See CCPM.

Foreign Unit Awards
See CCPM.

Non-U.S. Service Awards
See CCPM.

Association and Organization Awards
The order of precedence is as follows.
Commissioned Officers Association (of the USPHS, Inc.)
Association of Military Surgeons of the United States
Reserve Officers Association
Society of American Military Engineers

Ribbon Bars. Ribbons are worn in horizontal rows of three each. If not in multiples of three ribbons, the top row consists of the lesser number, with the center of this row located over the center of the row below it. The lower edge of the bottom row is centered ¼ inch above the left breast pocket. When the uppermost ribbons are covered by the coat lapel, the uppermost rows may contain two ribbons each, and aligned with the left border of the rack. Ribbons are arranged in the order of precedence in rows from the top down, and inboard to outboard within rows. All ribbons may be worn; if only one row of ribbons is worn, it must consist of the three senior ribbons.

Large Medals. Large medals are worn on Full Dress uniforms, suspended from a holding bar. Medals are worn in horizontal rows of three medals side by side, or up to five medals overlapping. Overlapping shall be equal, with the right or inboard medal showing in full. If not in equal multiples, all rows except the top row consist of equal numbers of medals and the top row consists of the lesser number of medals. Upper rows of medals are mounted so that these medals cover the suspension ribbons of the medals below. The medals are placed such that the bottom of each medal in a row constitutes a horizontal line. The lower edge of the bottom holding bar is centered ¼ inch above the left breast pocket. Medals are arranged in the order of precedence in rows from the top down, and inboard to outboard within rows. All medals may be worn; if only one row of medals is worn, it must consist of the five senior medals.

Miniature Medals. Miniature medals are worn with all Formal Dress uniforms and Dinner Dress uniforms, suspended from a holding bar. Medals are worn in horizontal rows of three to five medals side by side with no overlap. If not in equal multiples, all rows except the top row consist of equal numbers of medals and the top row consists of the lesser number of medals. Upper rows of medals are mounted so that these medals cover the suspension ribbons of the medals below. The medals are placed such that the bottom of each medal in a row constitutes a horizontal line. For Service Dress Blue or White coats, the lower edge of the bottom holding bar is centered ¼ inch above the left breast pocket. For the male officer's Formal and Dinner Dress jackets, the holding bar of the bottom row is positioned 3 inches below the notch and centered on the lapel. Three or more miniature medals are positioned starting at the inner edge of the lapel. For the female officer's Formal and Dinner Dress uniforms, the holding bar is worn in the same relative position as on the male's Dinner Dress jacket, down one-third of the distance from the shoulder seam to the coat hem. Medals are arranged in the order of precedence in rows from the top down, and inboard to outboard within rows. All medals may be worn; if only one row of medals is worn, it must consist of the five senior medals.

Ribbon and Medal Stars. Medal stars are worn on ribbons and medals in lieu of a second or subsequent like award. One or more stars are positioned in the center of the ribbon bar or the suspension ribbon of medals. When medals are worn overlapping, all stars may be positioned to the wearer's left.

For PHS Honor Awards, a 5/16" gold star is worn in lieu of a second like award, and a 5/16" silver star is worn in lieu of five gold stars. For PHS Unit and Service Awards, a 3/16" bronze star is worn in lieu of a second like award, and a 3/16" silver star is worn in lieu of five bronze stars. Stars are positioned such that one ray points up.

Standard Badges – Service Uniforms. The following badges and their placement on service uniforms are authorized:
- PHS Surgeon General (SG), Deputy Surgeon General (DSG), and Officer in Charge (OIC) insignia, full size, are placed on the officer's right side, centered just below the PHS name tag (females may alternatively relocate the badge above the name tag), while an incumbent of that position. Following completion of the tour of duty, the miniature badge is worn on the officer's left side, centered below the service ribbons or medals in the pocket area (females may relocate the miniature badge above the ribbons).
- PHS Recruiter or Associate Recruiter (AR) insignia, full size, are placed on the officer's left side, centered below the service ribbons in the left pocket area (females may relocate the badge above the name tag), and only while the officer has responsibility for or association with PHS recruitment programs. For males, the badge is 1 inch below the top of the pocket, or positioned midway between the pocket flap bottom and pocket bottom. For females, the uppermost portion of the badge either rests on or falls immediately below the pocket flap bottom; a badge worn centered above the PHS name tag is separated from the name tag by a ¼ to ⅜ inch space. The AR badge, when worn with a shirt as part of a Service uniform, may be suspended from the left pocket button by a plastic fob.
- Office of the Secretary of HHS Identification Badge (OSIB), is placed on the left breast pocket (females may relocate it above the name tag), and may be permanently worn upon completion of one continuous year of duty in a billet within the OS.
- Field Medical Readiness Badge (FMRB), silver, is worn on the left side, centered above the service ribbons.
- Authorized badges or breast insignia from other uniformed services are placed on the officer's left side, centered above the service ribbons.

Standard Badges – Ceremonial Uniforms. For ceremonial uniforms, standard badges are generally placed on the right pocket area, centered below all service, campaign and other ribbons authorized for which no large medals exist. Following completion of the SG, DSG or OIC tour of duty, the miniature badge is worn on the officer's left side, centered below the service ribbons or medals in the pocket area (females may alternatively relocate the miniature badge to the right side, above the ribbons authorized for which no large medals exist).

BASIC UNIFORM COMPONENTS, MALE

See the Commissioned Corps Personnel Manual for more information.

UNIFORM	COAT/JACKET	SHIRT	TROUSERS	SHOES	COMBINATION CAP	NECKTIE	BOARDS INSIGNIA	NAME TAG	DECORATIONS	NOTES
General Purpose Service Uniforms										
Service Dress Blue	Blue Dress	White	Blue Dress	Black	White	Black	-	Yes	Ribbons	1
Service Dress Blue Sweater	Black Army	White	Blue Dress	Black	White	Black	Soft Boards	Yes	-	1,2,3
Service Dress White	White Dress	-	White Dress	White	White	-	Hard Boards	Yes	Ribbons	
Service Blue (Salt & Pepper)	-	White SS	Blue	Black	White	-	Hard Boards	Yes	Ribbons	4
Service Khaki	-	Khaki SS	Khaki	Black	Khaki	-	Collar Insignia	Yes	Ribbons	5
Summer White	-	White SS	White	White	White	-	Hard Boards	Yes	Ribbons	6
Winter Blue	-	Blue LS	Blue	Black	White	Black	Collar Insignia	Yes	Ribbons	4
Working Uniforms										
Working Khaki	-	Khaki	Khaki	Black	Khaki	-	Collar Insignia	-	-	5,7
Indoor Duty White	-	White SS	White	White	White	-	Hard Boards	-	-	4,7
Winter Working Blue	-	Blue LS	Blue	Black	White	-	Collar Insignia	-	-	4,7
Special Situation Uniform										
Battle Dress Uniform	WCP Utility	-	WCP	Boots	-	-	Collar Insignia	-	-	8
Ceremonial Uniforms										
Full Dress Blue	Blue Dress	White LS	Blue Dress	Black	White	Black	-	-	Lge. Medals	9,10
Full Dress White	White Dress	-	White Dress	White	White	-	Hard Boards	-	Lge. Medals	9,10
Formal and Dinner Dress Uniforms										
Formal Dress	Blue Jacket	White Wing	Blue Evening	Black	-	White Bow	-	-	Min. Medals	11
Dinner Dress Blue Jacket	Blue Jacket	White TD	Blue Evening	Black	-	Black Bow	-	-	Min. Medals	12
Dinner Dress White Jacket	White Jacket	White TD	Blue Evening	Black	-	Black Bow	Hard Boards	-	Min. Medals	13
Dinner Dress Blue	Blue Dress	White LS	Blue Dress	Black	White	Black Bow	-	-	Min. Medals	14
Dinner Dress White	White Dress	-	White Dress	White	White	-	Hard Boards	-	Min. Medals	15
Tropical Dinner Dress Blue	-	White SS	Blue Dress	Black	White	-	Hard Boards	-	Min. Medals	16

Notes

1. Soft shoulder boards on shirt.
2. U.S. Army-style black, pullover, V-neck sweater.
3. Optional: Cap, blue garrison.
4. Optional/Prescribable: Cap, blue garrison; Jacket, black windbreaker; Sweater, black Army-style.
5. Optional/Prescribable: Cap, khaki garrison; Jacket, black or khaki windbreaker; Shoes, brown with khaki socks; Sweater, black Army-style.
6. Optional/Prescribable Items: Jacket, black windbreaker; Sweater, black Army-style.
7. Prescribable: PHS name tag.
8. Battle Dress Uniform (BDU). Woodland camouflage pattern (WCP). Required: WCP utility coat, with specified embroidered collar insignia, name and USPHS identification on olive green background; black crew neck undershirt, with specified PHS seal and U.S. Public Health Service print; WCP trousers with black web belt and black buckle; black combat boots; utility cap, with specified rank insignia.
9. Large medals/ribbons.
10. White gloves.
11. Formal Dress, equivalent to a white tie event. Jacket is Blue Dinner Dress; shirt is white wing collar; Mother of Pearl studs and cuff links; waistcoat; white gloves; use combination white cap with outer garment only.
12. Dinner Dress Blue Jacket, equivalent to a black tie event. Jacket is Blue Dinner Dress; shirt is white formal turndown, plain or with wide pleats; gold studs and cuff links; gold cummerbund; white gloves; use combination white cap with outer garment only.
13. Dinner Dress White Jacket, summertime equivalent to a black tie event. Jacket is White Dinner Dress; shirt is white formal turndown, plain or with wide pleats; gold studs and cuff links; gold cummerbund; white gloves; use combination white cap with outer garment only.
14. Dinner Dress Blue, as an option for a black tie event. Options include white formal turndown shirt; gold studs and cuff links; prescribable white gloves.
15. Dinner Dress White. Prescribable: White gloves.
16. Tropical Dinner Dress Blue. Gold wraparound cummerbund.

UNIFORMED SERVICE BASICS   27

BASIC UNIFORM COMPONENTS, FEMALE
See the Commissioned Corps Personnel Manual for more information.

UNIFORM	COAT/JACKET	SHIRT	SKIRT	SHOES	COMBINATION CAP	NECKTIE	BOARDS INSIGNIA	NAME TAG	DECORATIONS	NOTES
General Purpose Service Uniforms										
Service Dress Blue	Blue Dress	White	Blue Unbelted	Black	White	Black	-	Yes	Ribbons	1,2
Service Dress Blue Sweater	Black Army	White	Blue Unbelted	Black	White	Black	Soft Boards	Yes	-	1,2,3,4
Service Dress White	White Dress	White	White Unbelted	White	White	Black	-	Yes	Ribbons	1,5
Service Blue (Salt & Pepper)	-	White SS	Blue Belted	Black	White	-	Hard Board	Yes	Ribbons	6
Service Khaki	-	Khaki SS	Khaki Belted	Black	Khaki	-	Collar Insignia	Yes	Ribbons	7
Summer White	-	White SS	White Belted	White	White	-	Hard Boards	Yes	Ribbons	8
Winter Blue	-	Blue LS	Blue Belted	Black	White	Black	Collar Insignia	Yes	Ribbons	6
Working Uniforms										
Working Khaki	-	Khaki	Khaki Belted	Black	Khaki	-	Collar Insignia	-	-	7,9
Indoor Duty White	-	White SS	White Belted	White	White	-	Hard Boards	-	-	9,10
Winter Working Blue	-	Blue LS	Blue Belted	Black	White	-	Collar Insignia	-	-	6,9
Special Situation Uniforms										
Battle Dress Uniform	WCP Utility	-	WCP Trousers	Boots	-	-	Collar Insignia	-	-	11
Maternity Uniforms	*See Commissioned Corps Personnel Manual for information.*									
Ceremonial Uniforms										
Full Dress Blue	Blue Dress	White LS	Blue Unbelted	Black	White	Black	-	-	Lge. Medals	2,12,13
Full Dress White	White Dress	White LS	White Unbelted	White	White	Black	-	-	Lge. Medals	5,12,13
Formal and Dinner Dress Uniforms										
Formal Dress	Blue Jacket	White Dress	Blue Formal	Black Formal	-	Black Dress	-	-	Min. Medals	14
Dinner Dress Blue Jacket	Blue Jacket	White Dress	Blue Formal	Black Formal	-	Black Dress	-	-	Min. Medals	15
Dinner Dress White Jacket	White Jacket	White Dress	Blue Formal	Black Formal	-	Black Dress	-	-	Min. Medals	16
Dinner Dress Blue	Blue Dress	White LS	Blue Unbelted	Black	White	Black	-	-	Min. Medals	17
Dinner Dress White	White Dress	White LS	White Unbelted	White	White	Black	-	-	Min. Medals	18
Tropical Dinner Dress Blue	-	White SS	Blue Unbelted	Black	White	-	Hard Boards	-	Min. Medals	19

Notes

1. Soft shoulder boards on shirt.
2. Optional: Earrings, gold ball; Slacks, blue unbelted.
3. U.S. Army-style black, pullover, V-neck sweater.
4. Optional: Beret, black; Cap, blue garrison.
5. Optional: Earrings, gold ball; Slacks, white unbelted.
6. Optional/Prescribable: Beret, black; Cap, blue garrison; Earrings, gold ball; Jacket, black windbreaker; Slacks, blue belted; Sweater, black Army-style.
7. Optional/Prescribable: Cap, khaki garrison; Earrings, gold ball; Jacket, black or khaki windbreaker; Shoes, brown (with brown handbag); Slacks, khaki belted; Sweater, black Army-style.
8. Optional/Prescribable: Beret, black; Earrings, gold ball; Jacket, black windbreaker; Slacks, white belted.
9. Prescribable: PHS name tag.
10. Optional/Prescribable: Beret, black; Cap, blue garrison; Earrings, gold ball; Jacket, black windbreaker; Sweater, black Army-style.
11. Battle Dress Uniform (BDU). Woodland camouflage pattern (WCP). Required: WCP utility coat, with specified embroidered collar insignia, name and USPHS identification on olive green background; black crew neck undershirt, with specified PHS seal and U.S. Public Health Service print; WCP trousers with black web belt and black buckle; black combat boots; utility cap, with specified rank insignia.
12. Large medals/ribbons.
13. White gloves.
14. Formal Dress. Jacket is Blue Dinner Dress; shirt is white dress with tuxedo pleats; Mother of Pearl studs and cuff links; pearl earrings; skirt is long formal (blue formal slacks option); gold cummerbund; black dress handbag; white gloves; use combination white cap with outer garment only.
15. Dinner Dress Blue Jacket. Jacket is Blue Dinner Dress; shirt is white dress with tuxedo pleats; gold studs and cuff links; pearl earrings; skirt is long formal (blue formal slacks option); gold cummerbund; black dress handbag; white gloves; use combination white cap with outer garment only.
16. Dinner Dress White Jacket for summertime. Jacket is White Dinner Dress; shirt is white dress with tuxedo pleats; gold studs and cuff links; pearl earrings; skirt is long formal (blue formal slacks option); gold cummerbund; black dress handbag; white gloves; use combination white cap with outer garment only.
17. Dinner Dress Blue. Options include blue formal slacks; black formal shoes; gold studs and cuff links; pearl earrings; black dress handbag; white gloves.
18. Dinner Dress White. Options include white unbelted dress slacks; gold studs and cuff links; pearl earrings; black dress handbag; white gloves.
19. Tropical Dinner Dress Blue. Options include blue formal skirt or slacks; black formal shoes; pearl earrings; gold wraparound cummerbund; black dress handbag.

Section II.

Military Courtesy & Protocol

Each of the uniformed services has developed courtesies, customs and traditions that complement its legacy of service to the Nation. Such protocol and traditions are meant to enhance interpersonal relations and provide a heritage for future service personnel. Unlike traditions, however, the observance of standards of military protocol are required of all uniformed service personnel. PHS officers should be knowledgeable about, and render proper military courtesy at all times.

> ADDRESS & GREETING
> COMING TO ATTENTION
> FLAG ETIQUETTE
> HEADGEAR
> MILITARY FUNERAL
> POSITION OF HONOR
> SALUTING

Address & Greeting

Use of Titles
Uniformed service personnel are properly addressed by their military rank and surname or, if appropriate, by rank. Titles of military rank consist of two groups:
- Titles of rank are the same for personnel in the U.S. Coast Guard, Navy, National Oceanic and Atmospheric Administration (NOAA), and Public Health Service; and
- Titles of rank are the same for commissioned personnel in the U.S. Air Force, Army, and Marine Corps, but differ for enlisted personnel among these services.

U.S. Coast Guard, Navy, NOAA, PHS

Enlisted Personnel. The term *rate* refers to the rank of Navy enlisted personnel. The rate, or grade, always precedes an enlisted person's surname. A chief petty officer is addressed as "Chief," "Senior Chief" or "Master Chief." Chief warrant officers may be addressed as "Mister" or "Ms."

Commissioned Officers. The rank always precedes an officer's surname. In conversation and greetings (cf., written communication), titles of commissioned officers are as follows:

- All commanders—lieutenant commander and commander—are addressed as "Commander." Coast Guard and Navy officers below the rank of commander may be addressed as "Mr. (surname)" or "Ms. (surname)" during routine duty, although this convention is no longer specified by regulation.
- All admirals—rear, vice, admiral, and fleet admiral—are addressed "Admiral."

By custom, the officer who commands a ship is addressed as "Captain" (or "Skipper") regardless of his rank. Similarly, the executive officer of a ship is addressed as "Commander," and may be referred to as the "Executive Officer" or "XO." The USPHS commanding officer is the Surgeon General who is addressed as "Surgeon General (surname)" or "Admiral."

U.S. Air Force, Army, Marine Corps

Enlisted Personnel. The military grade, or rank, always precedes an enlisted soldier's surname. A warrant officer, however, ranks just below a second lieutenant and is addressed as "Mister" or "Ms.," and those above the rank of warrant officer (W-1) in less formal circumstances are addressed as "Chief."

Commissioned Officers. The rank always precedes an officer's surname. In conversation and greetings (cf., written communication), titles of commissioned officers are as follows:

- All lieutenants—first and second lieutenants—are addressed "Lieutenant."
- All colonels—lieutenant colonel and colonel—are addressed "Colonel."
- All generals—brigadier, major, lieutenant, and general—are addressed as "General."

By custom, the head of an Air Force, Army or Marine Corps base or unit is referred to as "the Commanding Officer" or "CO."

All Uniformed Services

Subordinate personnel address a superior as "Sir" or "Ma'am," by rank, or by rank and surname. The superior officer addresses a subordinate, whether a commissioned officer or an enlisted service member, by rank, or by rank and surname. In informal work circumstances, officers will usually address each other by their given names. When in formal situations or when outside personnel are present, officers should use prescribed forms of address.

In all branches of the uniformed services, a descriptive title may be used instead of rank for certain officers. For example, officers in the dental and medical professions may be addressed as "Doctor" regardless of rank (except for flag officers, who are always addressed as "Admiral"). Clergy may be addressed as "Chaplain" regardless of rank or religion. During official introductions, however, these officers' ranks should be used.

The following table shows the equivalent titles of rank for commissioned officers at each pay grade.

MILITARY TITLES OF RANK
COMMISSIONED OFFICERS

PAY GRADE	NAVY/COAST GUARD NOAA/PHS	ARMY	AIR FORCE MARINE CORPS
01	Ensign ENS	Second Lieutenant 2LT	Second Lieutenant 2nd Lt.
02	Lieutenant Jr Grade LTJG	First Lieutenant 1LT	First Lieutenant 1st Lt.
03	Lieutenant LT	Captain CPT	Captain Capt.
04	Lieutenant Commander, LCDR	Major MAJ	Major Maj.
05	Commander CDR	Lieutenant Colonel LTC	Lieutenant Colonel Lt. Col.
06	Captain CAPT	Colonel COL	Colonel Col.
07	Rear Admiral Lower Half, RADM (LH)	Brigadier General BG	Brigadier General Brig. Gen.
08	Rear Admiral Upper Half, RADM *Director, NOAA Corps*	Major General MG	Major General Maj. Gen.
09	Vice Admiral VADM *Surgeon General, PHS*	Lieutenant General LTG	Lieutenant General Lt. Gen.
10	Admiral ADM *Assistant Secretary for Health, PHS* *Chief of Naval Operations* *Commandant of the Coast Guard*	General GEN *Army Chief of Staff*	General Gen. *Air Force Chief of Staff* *Commandant of the Marine Corps*
11	Fleet Admiral FADM [Wartime only]	General of the Army [Wartime only]	General of the Air Force [Wartime only]

Handshake
When situations call for shaking hands, the subordinate service member should wait until the senior officer offers his/her hand. When gloves are prescribed, you can remove your right glove, time permitting, when being introduced outdoors; when indoors, remove both gloves. The proper way to shake hands is to keep your hand in a vertical plane, extending your hand with the thumb up and fingers pointed outward. The two hands connect "web to web" in a comfortably firm, solid grip. Shake with two or three smooth hand pumps.

Coming to Attention

The position of attention is a military courtesy, and is the basic military stance that indicates a person is alert and ready. The position of attention is also the pre-position for facing and marching movements.

When to be at Attention
Subordinate personnel in uniform come to attention in prescribed situations. PHS officers should assume the position of attention in certain circumstances:
- When called to attention by the officer in charge.
- When rendering a salute *(see the Section "Saluting")*.
- When being formally spoken to by a senior officer.
- While the national anthem is being played indoors (no salute).
- When an officer of superior rank enters a room and the command is given, "Attention" or "Attention on Deck." Alternatively, the junior officer who first sees the superior officer announces, for example, "Ladies and Gentlemen, the Surgeon General!" at which all officers stand at attention. The room is not called to attention when an officer of equal or higher rank is already in the room. Unless entering the room for the purpose of addressing the group, the superior officer promptly responds, "As You Were."

How to Stand at Attention
Stand and assume the position of attention by bringing the heels together on line with the feet pointing out equally, forming a 45-degree angle. Rest the weight of the body equally on the heels and balls of the feet. Keep the legs straight without stiffening or locking the knees. Hold the body erect with the hips level, stomach in, chest lifted and arched, and the shoulders square and even.

Let the arms hang straight without stiffness. With the hands turned inward, curl the fingers so that the tips of the thumbs are alongside and touching the first joint of the forefingers. Keep the thumbs straight along the seams of the trouser legs (for a skirt, the lateral mid-point of the thigh), with fingers touching the legs. The head is held erect and square, facing straight to the front, with the chin drawn in so that the alignment of the head and neck is vertical.

Flag Etiquette

The United States Code is the official compilation of Federal laws currently in force. The Code is divided into 50 titles by subject matter, with Title 4, Chapter 1 and Title 36, Chapter 10 being the primary laws that govern the handling and display of the U.S. flag. The terms flag, color, standard, or ensign may be used to designate the national flag. The *national color* is carried by dismounted units, such as a color guard. The *standard* refers to the national flag when mounted on vehicles. The *ensign* is the term used for the national flag when flown from ships.

Raising and Lowering the Flag

Morning colors (Naval term) or reveille (Army, Air Force) is the daily ceremony of raising the national flag, and evening colors or retreat is the ceremony of lowering the national flag. The national flag is raised briskly and lowered ceremoniously. Although normally displayed only between sunrise and sunset, it may be displayed during the hours of darkness if properly illuminated. Uniformed service personnel come to attention and render a salute while the flag is hoisted or lowered, with the salute held until the last note of the music or bugle call, or the flag is unsnapped from the halyard, whichever is longer.

Displaying the Flag

There are numerous rules for displaying the flag and those which follow are most pertinent to uniformed services.

Indoors. When the U.S. flag is displayed indoors with other flags, it is placed in the position of honor, which is to the flag's own right (i.e., the observer's left), with all other flags arranged to the left of the U.S. flag in decreasing order of precedence. No other flag or pennant should be placed to the right or above the U.S. flag. For uniformed service receptions and dinners, it is customary to display the national color and other flags in a "flag line" that is centered behind the receiving line or head table. When a podium is used, the U.S. flag is placed to the right of the staging area in advance of the audience, and other flags to the left of the speaker (Figure 1).

The U.S. flag is centered and its staff placed vertically at the highest point among a number of flags of states or localities or pennants grouped and displayed from staffs. When the U.S. flag is displayed with another flag where staffs are crossed, the U.S. flag is placed on its own right with its staff positioned in front of the staff of the other flag (Figure 2).

If displayed flat against a wall (indoors or outdoors), either horizontally or vertically, the flag's union (stars) is positioned at the top and to the flag's own right (Figure 3).

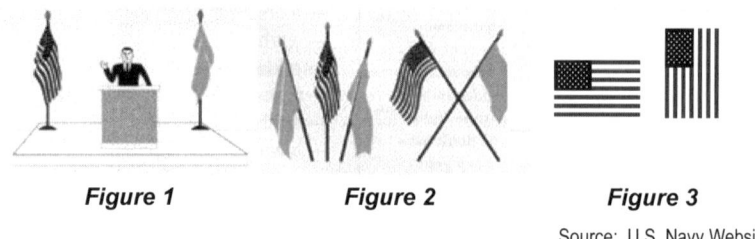

| Figure 1 | Figure 2 | Figure 3 |

Source: U.S. Navy Website

Outdoors. When displayed outdoors, the U.S. flag is always positioned at the top of the flagpole when other flags are flown on the same pole. When separate flag poles are used for the national flag with other flags, the U.S. flag is placed in the position of honor, to its own right; the other flags may be the same size, but not larger than the U.S. flag, nor may other flags be placed higher than the U.S. flag; and, the U.S. flag is always the first to be raised and the last to be lowered.

When flown with flags of other nations, each flag should be approximately the same size and displayed on a separate pole of the same height. All flags are raised and lowered simultaneously.

When displayed on a car, the U.S. flag staff is affixed firmly to the chassis or clamped to the front right fender.

Parading the Flag
In procession, the national flag is always accorded the place of honor, which is the position to its own right (i.e., the viewer's left). When carried with another flag(s), the U.S. flag is positioned to its own right or, if there is a line of other flags, it may be carried in front of the center of that line. When the flag passes in procession, uniformed personnel face the flag and salute at that moment, whereas those in formation salute upon command of the officer in charge. Persons not in uniform place their right hand over their heart, and men with a hat remove it with their right hand and hold it at the left shoulder with the hand being over their heart.

The Flag in Mourning
Only the President of the United States or a state governor can order the U.S. flag be lowered to half-staff (*half-mast* in the Navy). When flown at half-staff, the U.S. flag is first hoisted to the peak for an instant and then lowered to a position one-half the distance between the top and bottom of the staff. The flag is again raised to the peak before being lowered for the day. On Memorial Day, the U.S. flag is displayed at half-staff until noon, at which time it is raised to full staff.

When used to cover a casket, the U.S. flag is placed with the union at the head and over the left shoulder. The flag should not touch the ground and it is not lowered into the grave.

The National Anthem and Pledge of Allegiance

When the national anthem is played or sung outdoors, uniformed personnel stand at attention and render a salute to the flag at the first note of the anthem, and hold the salute to the last note. When the flag is not displayed or not in view, uniformed personnel face toward the music. During recitation of the pledge of allegiance outdoors, uniformed personnel remain silent, stand at attention and hold a salute to the flag. Persons not in uniform place their right hand over their heart during the national anthem and pledge of allegiance.

Folding the Flag

There is a traditional method for folding the United States flag *(see Figures)*.

Step 1. Two persons hold the flag parallel to the ground, waist-high. Fold the lower striped half of the flag over the blue field of stars.

Step 2. Fold the flag again lengthwise—begin with the folded edge and bring it up to meet the open edges, with the blue field on the outside.

Step 3. A triangular fold is started by bringing the striped corner of the folded edge to meet the open edge of the flag. Then turn the outer point inward, parallel with the open edge, to form a second triangle. The triangular folding is continued until the length of the flag is folded in this manner and only the blue field is visible.

Step 4. Fold down the square into a triangle and tuck inside the folds.

Folding the U.S. flag will take thirteen folds: two lengthwise folds and eleven triangular folds.

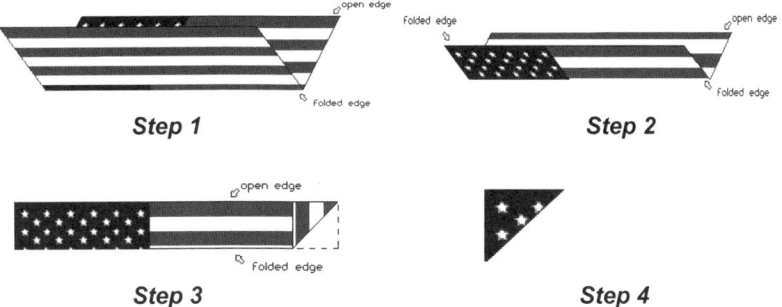

Headgear

When wearing the uniform outdoors, the cap, also referred to as the cover, is always worn and never removed or raised as a form of salutation. The cap need not be worn outside in an area designated by the local commander as a "covered area." For example, a covered area could be the transit area between a group of buildings. For safety reasons, caps are to be removed and secured upon entering an active aircraft landing area, airfield tarmac or helicopter landing zone.

Generally, personnel remove their cover when entering a building and remain uncovered while indoors. However, officers may remain covered in a public building such as an airport.

Military Funeral

The provision of Military Funeral Honors is based on custom and tradition. The ceremony is carried out with dignity and respect, as a display of the Nation's gratitude for those men and women who have served our Country. Burial in a national cemetery (other than Arlington National Cemetery) is generally provided to PHS officers who have served on active duty and were separated under other than dishonorable conditions. Military honors may be provided at the time of burial, depending on the status of the deceased and the availability of uniformed service personnel.

Elements of the Ceremony
The military funeral has certain basic elements that are common to all such ceremonies. For eligible *veterans,* the core elements of the funeral honors ceremony will be performed, consisting of the ceremonial folding and presentation of the American flag and sounding of Taps (bugler or a quality recording). At least two uniformed service persons and a bugler, if available, shall perform the ceremony. One of the uniformed personnel is a representative of the Public Health Service and shall present the flag to the family. Uniformed services are encouraged to provide additional elements of honors as personnel and resources permit.

For members who die while on *active duty,* the honors detail may consist of an officer-in-charge (OIC, who may be the officer representing the PHS), six uniformed body bearers (casket team), a seven-person firing detail and a bugler. When personnel are limited, funeral honors can be efficiently rendered by a detail of the OIC and eight members, who serve as both the body bearers and firing detail.

In addition, up to eight honorary pallbearers may be selected by family of the deceased. Honorary pallbearers form two facing ranks, such that the casket is carried between the two ranks when it is brought into and out of a chapel, and when the casket is moved from the hearse (or caisson at Arlington National Cemetery) to the burial lot. When marching, the honorary pallbearers form two columns on each side of the hearse.

Flags. American flags are provided for burial services of service members and veterans. The flag for those who die on active duty is provided by the PHS, and the flag for veterans is provided by the Department of Veterans Affairs.

Sequence of Events. The general sequence of Military Funeral Honors, beginning with a chapel service, is as follows.
- The immediate family, relatives and friends of the deceased are seated in the chapel before the casket is carried in.
- The honorary pallbearers take positions in two facing ranks in front of the chapel entrance before the hearse arrives. Upon arrival, the honorary pallbearers execute the hand salute when the body bearers remove the casket from the hearse.
- The body bearers then carry the casket, foot end first (reverse for a chaplain's funeral), between the two ranks. The honorary pallbearers come to the order and fall in behind the casket as it is carried into the chapel. In the chapel, the honorary pallbearers take places in the left front pews and the casket team in the rear pews *(see illustration below)*.

Chapel Formation

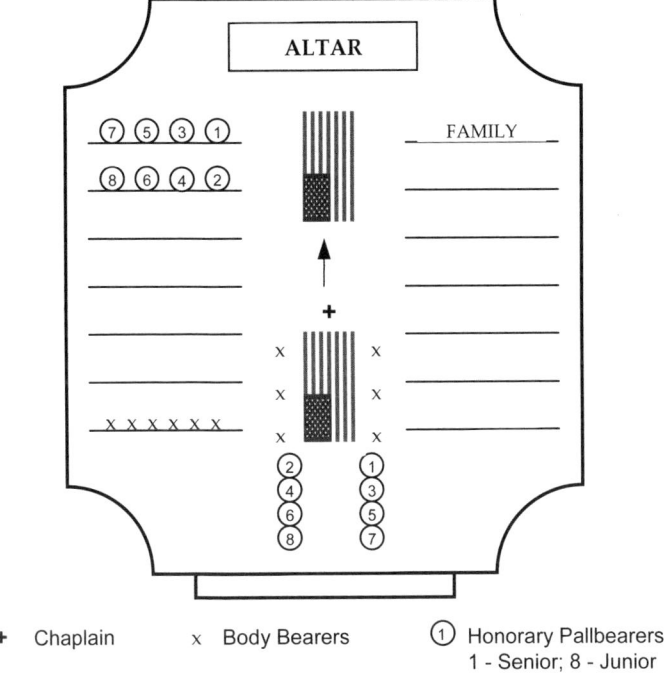

+ Chaplain   x Body Bearers   ① Honorary Pallbearers
1 - Senior; 8 - Junior

- After the chapel service, the reverse order is followed: the honorary pallbearers precede the casket in two columns and, just outside the chapel entrance, form two facing ranks between which the casket is carried to the hearse.

- The casket is covered with the American flag and transported to, and within the cemetery in the hearse.
- Upon reaching the grave site, the casket is secured and carried by the body bearers. The casket is placed over the grave and the casket team holds the flag, stretched out and level, waist high over the casket throughout the service.
- After the committal service is read by the chaplain, the OIC presents arms to initiate three rifle volleys.
- A bugler sounds Taps. The flag is folded by the casket team and the head body bearer passes the flag to the OIC and then salutes. The casket team departs. The OIC either presents the flag to the family, or hands the flag to the chaplain who then presents it to the family. The flag is presented with appropriate condolences; for example, "On behalf of a grateful Nation and a proud Public Health Service, I present this flag to you in recognition of your (relationship)'s years of honorable and faithful service to his/her Country." The presenter will then step back one pace and render the hand salute.

The military funeral is completed.

Military Salutes

All uniformed personnel attending in their individual capacity salute the caisson or hearse when it arrives at the cemetery. Render the hand salute at any time when the casket is being moved, while the casket is being lowered into the grave, during the firing of the volley, and while Taps is being sounded.

Position of Honor

The position of honor is always to the right. Thus, junior officers ride, sit, or walk to the left of senior officers. The place of honor in an automobile is the right rear seat, although some senior officers prefer to sit in the front passenger seat. When entering the rear seat of an automobile from the right side, officers enter in inverse order of rank, allowing the senior officer to enter last and sit on the right; the senior then is the first to disembark. Alternatively, safety permitting, the junior officer will open and close the right rear door for the senior officer, and the junior officer will enter through the left rear door. If three officers are in the rear seat, the junior officer sits in the middle; alternatively, the junior officer should move to the front passenger seat if unoccupied.

When there is a head table at a meeting or official function, the place of honor is to the right of the chairperson or host or the center podium. Senior officers are also accorded the most desirable seats in all settings. A junior officer should open a door to allow the senior officer to enter first, and then pass through after the senior officer.

Saluting

The military salute has an uncertain origin. It may be related to the knights in armor who used their right hand (their left hand held the horse reins) to raise their visor to identify themselves and as a gesture of friendship. Today, the right hand salute is a gesture of greeting and respect among service personnel. It is rendered to all uniformed service commissioned and warrant officers, the President of the United States, senior U.S. government officials, any Medal of Honor recipient, and officers of friendly foreign countries.

Forms of Salute
An officer normally uses the hand salute. If under arms, render the salute prescribed for the weapon with which armed. When entering a military installation, an officer may receive a rifle salute by the gate guard; this is returned with a hand salute.

The sword or saber salute involves bringing the hilt to the chin, the flat of the blade opposite to the right eye, sword point up, and a subsequent lowering of the point to the ground until the person to whom the salute is rendered has passed six paces.

Cannon salutes are reserved to honor high civilian and military officials. The number of cannon blasts is prescribed according to the honored person's rank.

Hand Salute Basics
Both an initial hand salute and a return hand salute are required. The salute is always initiated by a person of junior rank, whether enlisted or officer, to an officer who is senior in rank. The initiating salute is held until after a return salute or acknowledgement is made by the higher ranking officer. When rendering a salute, one's head and eyes are turned to the person being saluted or to the Colors.

If *standing,* the junior officer salutes from the position of attention. When *walking,* the salute should be initiated in sufficient time to allow a response by the senior officer; the general guide is to initiate a salute between six and 30 paces. It is courteous to accompany one's salute with a verbal greeting to the senior officer such as "Good morning (afternoon, evening), Sir/Ma'am." Upon saluting, the senior officer should similarly reply with the subordinate's rank ("Good morning, Lieutenant"). If two officers or an officer and enlisted member approach one another with the intent of conversing, salutes are exchanged upon meeting and again after the conversation, before departing.

How to Salute
The hand salute is performed by raising the right hand smartly, fingers extended and joined, palm down and slightly turned toward the face. The hand is brought upward until the tip of the forefinger/middle finger touches the right

front corner of the headdress; if wearing a nonbilled cap, touch the forehead slightly to the right and above the right eye or the right front corner of eyeglasses. Hold the upper arm horizontal with the elbow slightly forward, the forearm inclined at an angle, and the hand and wrist straight. To complete the salute, the hand is dropped smartly to the position of attention at one's side.

When to Salute
Personnel in uniform and with head cover are required to render salutes in the following instances.
- When approaching a senior officer in uniform.
- When saluted by junior officers or enlisted personnel.
- When passing a senior officer who is walking in the same direction, the subordinate holds a salute when abreast stating, "By your leave, Sir/Ma'am;" the senior officer returns the salute with "Carry On."
- Upon the command, "Present, Arms."
- To the national color (U.S. flag mounted on a flagstaff with finial) outdoors, holding the salute six steps distance before until six steps after it passes by, or before and after passing it.
- At morning and evening colors (same as reveille and retreat), when the national flag is being raised or lowered. Personnel face the flag or, if not visible, face in the direction of the flag and/or music and hold the salute from the first note of "Reveille." Note that in the evening, the bugle call "Retreat" is first sounded and all personnel come to attention; following that, the national anthem or "To the Colors" is played during which all personnel render and hold a salute until the music has finished.
- During the playing of the U.S. national anthem, the bugle call "To the Colors," "Hail to the Chief," or a foreign national anthem.
- When flag rank officers within official vehicles pass by.
- When the Pledge of Allegiance is recited at civilian events outdoors.
- During the sounding of honors.
- On ceremonial occasions (e.g., command change, military parades).
- When turning over control of formations.

When Saluting is Not Required
- When officers of equal rank approach each other (optional salute).
- When impractical, such as carrying packages in both hands.
- When either the subordinate or senior member is wearing civilian clothes (optional salute).
- When at large public gatherings such as sporting events.
- Indoors; in a "covered" area; and, when the national anthem is played indoors (military personnel stand at attention).

In all of these instances (not including the national anthem), a nod or verbal greeting (preferred) is proper.

Other Situations
Formation. When an individual is in charge of a formation or work detail, he salutes for the group. Formation members do not salute except at the command of the ranking officer. If not already at attention, the commands are as follows: "Attention;" personnel salute at "Present, Arms" or "Hand, Salute," and complete the salute after the command "Order, Arms" or "Ready, Two."

Military Installations. An officer entering a military post may receive a rifle salute by an enlisted person under arms serving as a guard. This is a salute to the officer and should be returned as if it were a hand salute. While driving on a military base, vehicles should stop and occupants disembark to salute the flag when colors are sounded.

Reporting (pertains to the Armed Forces). If formally reporting to a commanding officer in his/her office, a certain procedure is followed. Upon reaching the office, an officer removes his cover, knocks, and enters the room when called. The service member approaches the officer's desk and stops about two paces away. Come to attention and render a hand salute stating, "Sir/Ma'am, (your rank, first and last name) reporting." For example, "Ma'am, Lieutenant Robert Smith reporting."

Ship Boarding. When boarding a commissioned vessel of a uniformed service, uniformed personnel should stop at the top of the gangway, turn toward the ship's stern and salute the ensign. Then, turn to face and salute the officer of the deck (OOD, who may be a commissioned, warrant or senior petty officer). While saluting, state the request "Sir/Ma'am, I request permission to come aboard," setting foot on deck only after the salute is returned and permission is granted. If appropriate, you will say "(your rank and name) reporting for duty, Sir/Ma'am." On leaving the ship, face and salute the OOD and state that you have permission to go ashore (enlisted persons request permission to leave). When the OOD returns the salute and/or grants permission, walk a few steps, turn and salute the aft ensign, and then disembark.

SECTION III.

CEREMONIAL & SOCIAL PROTOCOL

Commissioned officers will, at various times throughout their career, plan and participate in official ceremonies and social functions. These formal events are important in building a sense of community within the service. Social activities, whether associated with a uniformed service or civilian life, provide a social fabric that helps to bond people in friendship. In this section, those social activities identified with military life are discussed. These functions are based on custom and tradition, and it is important that officers familiarize themselves with the basic protocol of such events.

> DINING-IN & DINING-OUT
> OFFICIAL DINNERS & RECEPTIONS
> PRESENTATION OF AWARDS
> PROMOTION CEREMONY
> RETIREMENT CEREMONY

Dining-In & Dining-Out

The dining-in and dining-out are formal dinners that are a tradition in all of the uniformed services. It is thought that dining-in had its inception in antiquity, beginning with the early Roman legions, Vikings, and English knights who held great feasts to celebrate victories in battle and individual feats of heroism. Formalized dining-in is also thought to have been a practice in old English monastic life. The monks, as educators, spread the custom to universities where graduates, who later became British officers, may have carried the tradition to the military. The British "guest night" was adopted by the early Continental Army and Navy of the U.S., and slowly took hold within the U.S. armed services. While often used for special occasions such as welcoming new officers or recognizing a dignitary, these ceremonial dinners are primarily a social occasion to pay tribute and promote good fellowship among officers.

Dining-In
The dining-in as practiced in the Navy and Air Force is also known as mess night in the Marine Corps and Coast Guard, and regimental dinner in the Army. A dining-in is held by a military unit or organization for its own officers *only*. For many years, it was considered a command function at which all officers of the command were expected to be present. In recent years, attendance at the dining-in is encouraged, but deemed voluntary.

Dining-Out
The dining-out is similar to dining-in, but is inclusive of service members' spouses, personal guests and invited members of other uniformed services. Officers of the sponsoring unit are the "members of the mess," and all others attend by invitation. Dining-in/dining-out, hereinafter referred to as dining-out, are formal events that are at the same time intended to be spirited and enjoyed by all participants.

Dress
Uniformed service dress for the occasion is the Dinner Dress Blue Jacket or Dinner Dress White Jacket, without gloves (prescribable). Lieutenants and below may wear Dinner Dress Blue or Dinner Dress White (Service Dress Blue/White with black bow tie and miniature medals, no name tag). Civilian dress is tuxedo or business suit for men, and formal or cocktail dress without gloves for women.

Elements
The format and program sequence of the dining-out varies among services, but the PHS tends to follow the Navy model with modifications. The dining-out is planned well in advance to ensure a successful program. Principal elements of the function are a formal setting such as the officers' club, a fine dinner, traditional toasts, presence of honored guests and camaraderie of the members.

The dining-out has a presiding senior officer or president, assisted by an officer serving in the capacity of a vice-president called "Mister/Madame Vice" (or, "the Vice"). Mr. Vice should be witty and is the only person allowed to speak without the president's leave. In addition, the occasion usually has an honored guest who is an official guest seated at the head table. The president, honored/distinguished guests and their spouses sit at a head table on one side only, facing the attendees. Mr. Vice sits at a small table away from the head table, where he can view the president and also observe the entire room. The president uses a gavel to direct attendees, as follows: one rap means be seated, two raps mean rise, and three raps mean attention.

Reception
The pre-dinner reception allows members and guests to meet one another, and provides an opportunity to greet the official guests and senior officers. It is important that members and their guests arrive on time for this activity which is considered integral to the event purpose.

Dinner
When it is time for the dinner, a chime is sounded or a bagpiper, if available, plays marching music and leads the group into the mess (dining area). Members and guests should not carry drinks to the mess. Diners stand quietly behind their chairs, at which time the head table officers and guests enter. When those at the head table are in place, the music ceases. The president calls the mess to order and directs the Surgeon General's Honor Corps. The PHS Music Ensemble leads the group in singing the national anthem and the PHS March. The president then raps the gavel once and invites everyone to be seated. The president will at this time make a few opening remarks, to include welcoming guests of the mess and introducing the guest of honor and principal officers of the event. Dinner commences after the following two rituals are accomplished.

Inspection of the Beef. The piper will play "Roast Beef of Olde England" as the president or other designee marches over to sample the beef entrée. If acceptable, the president announces to the diners that "The beef is fit for human consumption."

Mixing of the Grog. The president or designee will next describe the flavorful (nonalcoholic) ingredients of the grog, which are then mixed together.

Violations of the Mess Rules
The organizers of a dining-out will prepare "rules of the mess," which are often laced with humor, and include them in the printed program. Once the dinner begins, penalties will be levied for violations of rules of the mess. During the meal, members are encouraged to note violations by other members of the mess; this is done by raising a point of order with Mr. Vice. The president or Mr. Vice may allow an accused offender the opportunity to rebut the charges, and will render a judgment on the validity of the charge. Infractions are noted and penalties levied for said offenses. The usual penalty is a small fine, the proceeds of which are sent to a charity or used for a special purpose. A member who is in violation of the rules must pay a fine and drink from the grog bowl. Upon reaching the grog bowl, the member should salute the president, fill a cup, toast the mess ("To the Mess"), drain the contents of the cup, place the cup upside down (indicating it is empty), and again salute the president before returning to his/her seat.

Recess
When the dinner is finished, the president raps the gavel three times to get everyone's attention, and announces a short recess for participants to refresh themselves and to allow the wait staff to remove all dishes, flatware and glasses. The gavel is then rapped twice, indicating that members should stand and wait by their chairs until the head table has departed. This also signals that the program relating to rule violations is concluded.

When the recess is over, members will be led by the piper back to the mess, where they should remain standing behind their chairs until the head table has made their entry and the president invites everyone to be seated.

Wine Pouring
When the table is cleared, the wait staff will place wine glasses and decanters of wine (port wine is traditional) on the dining tables. Each person fills his/her own glass with wine. By custom, the decanter is passed only to the right around the table, without touching the table, until all glasses are filled (charged). The most junior officer at each table is responsible for ensuring that all glasses are charged. Those who prefer not to drink an alcoholic beverage can choose to fill their glass with wine but not sip from it during the toast, or they may drink water or other nonalcoholic beverage (not soda) with which to toast.

Toasts
Formal. At this time, the president begins formal toasts to the positions held by high ranking officials, honored guests, and to institutions. Traditionally, the president starts by standing and offering a toast to the President of the United States (known as the Loyalty Toast). The president or vice president may also toast the Surgeon General. For example, the president will state, "To the Surgeon General of the United States." Mr. Vice stands and seconds the toast, "Gentlemen, Ladies, the Surgeon General of the United States." Diners should rise (non-military women remain seated), repeat the toast in unison, "The Surgeon General" while raising their glasses, and take a sip of wine. Thereafter, the president may recognize members who offer pre-arranged formal toasts, including toasts to each professional category. Protocol is that a toast by the president is seconded by Mr. Vice and a toast by a member of the mess is seconded by the president.

Informal. The president then will invite members of the mess to offer informal toasts—these may be humorous (in good taste). An officer must rise and first request to propose a toast from Mr. Vice. When recognized, the officer proceeds with the toast. If deemed suitable, the president seconds the toast. All present should respond to this and subsequent informal toasts with "Hear, Hear!"

Honored Guest Address
The president reintroduces the guest of honor, who will address the group for about 10 to 15 minutes on a topic that is entertaining or uplifting and consistent with the intent of the dining-out. Following the address, Mr. Vice may propose a toast to the guest speaker.

Cake Ceremony
In the PHS, a cake (preferably bearing the U.S. Public Health Service logo), after being properly inspected, is cut with a PHS sword by the honored guest and most junior officer present and served to all present.

Concluding Activities
The president will conclude the evening with a final, formal toast to the U.S. Public Health Service (if not earlier offered). Mr. Vice faces the mess and seconds the toast. All present rise, repeat the toast in unison, "The United States Public Health Service," and drain their glasses. Everyone should remain standing at their places while the PHS March music is played. The president will then thank the guest of honor and other guests for their attendance and key organizers of the event. Those at the head table will then depart the mess, followed by members and guests.

Planning
Planning and preparations for a dining-out should begin three to four months in advance of the event date. For those officers tasked with planning a dining-out, a planning checklist is provided in Appendix A.

Official Dinners & Receptions

The military services have traditionally been strongly supportive of social functions as a way to enhance the lives of its members. These occasions build a sense of community, and are particularly important because officers and their families are often assigned to a duty station for only three or four years, and they may be at a remote duty station or live on a military base where civilian socializing is limited.

Official social functions range from informal to formal affairs. Less formal occasions include functions such as "hails and farewells" to welcome newcomers and bid farewell to those leaving a duty station. Formal dinners and receptions are usually held to honor someone or mark a special occasion. Truly formal events that call for engraved invitations are infrequent.

Official PHS functions are conducted in much the same way as in civilian society, and officers are expected to know the rules of social etiquette. Officers will have occasion to be invited to these functions and may even participate in planning such an event. The information which follows covers those topics which may pertain to semi-formal and formal functions.

Basics

Some basic guidance is provided for those attending social functions. For more detailed information, see the Section entitled *Table Protocol*.

Be on Time. For receptions with a receiving line, one should arrive within 20 minutes of the starting time or before the receiving line disbands. For formal dinners, it is essential to arrive on time and preferably before the starting time.

Consuming Food. When hors d'oeuvres are served, avoid standing around the buffet table for long periods of time, so as not to give the appearance of being wedded to the food and to allow easy access to the table by others.

Conversation. Senior officers at a reception should make an effort to converse with junior officers, including those not known. When at a dining table, it is important to talk with those who are seated on both sides of you.

Departures. It is no longer improper to leave before a guest of honor, but it is important to greet an honored guest or ranking official before leaving.

Seating. Seating at formal dinners may be by order of precedence or assigned. Ensure that seating is not prearranged before taking your place. Due deference should be given by junior officers to those more senior, allowing senior officers to sit at preferred locations at the table, if applicable.

Invitations

Generally, invitations are extended about three to four weeks before the event. Invitations to large or important affairs, or to functions planned during a holiday season, should be sent at least one month in advance.

Types and Content of Invitations. There are several accepted ways to extend an invitation. For informal and semi-formal occasions, invitations may be extended in the following ways: given in person; by telephone; e-mail for large, informal gatherings; "fill-in" preprinted card; handwritten card; or by a printed card.

For formal occasions, invitations may be extended in the following ways: by telephone, followed by a "To Remind" card; handwritten card; thermographed (raised print) card; or by engraved card. An engraved card is used only for the most formal occasions, with white or cream color cardstock and matching envelopes.

All written invitations should contain complete information about the function. When the occasion calls for a printed or engraved invitation, the text is normally written in the third person. Information is usually centered and, starting at the top, includes the following *(see the Sample Invitation on page 49):*

- *Who*—the host of the function, either an organization or individual. Ranks and names are written in full. For very high ranking officials, the position title is used (e.g., The Surgeon General). An admiral's flag may be centered at the top or the upper left corner of his/her invitations.

Follow with a phrase such as "cordially invites you" or, when also intended for one's spouse, the phrase "requests the company of" is used.

- *What*—the type of function, such as "at a reception." If more than one activity is planned, indicate that here or in the lower right corner.
- *Why*—the purpose, such as "in honor of."
- *When*—the day, date of the week and time; the day, date (no year) and hour are spelled out, with the day and month capitalized.
- *Where*—the name and address of the venue and, if applicable, the name of the banquet or meeting room.
- *Dress*—if not evident from the event, the dress code is provided in the lower right corner.
- *How to Reply*—RSVP is the abbreviation for répondez s'il vous plaît, meaning please reply. The RSVP is located in the lower left corner of the invitation, and will include the contact information. The invitation may also specify "Regrets Only." Alternatively, a RSVP card and self-addressed return envelope may be enclosed.

Mailing Invitations. Invitations are inserted into the envelope so that the text faces the back side of the envelope and the top coincides with the top of the envelope. Secondary materials, such as a RSVP card, are placed behind the invitation (or inside a double fold invitation) within the envelope. Envelope addresses may be typed or handwritten (do not use labels). For formal events, envelopes should only be handwritten in black ink.

Replies. Respond promptly regarding your acceptance of an invitation; normally, this should be done within 48 hours of receiving an invitation.

Canceling an Acceptance. There are few acceptable reasons for not showing or canceling after accepting an invitation. A cancellation of your initial acceptance should be briefly explained, with a sincere apology. Cancellations should be telephoned as soon as possible and, for very important functions, followed with a written note.

Sample Invitation

> The Commissioned Officers Association
> of the U.S. Public Health Service
> cordially invites you to
> a dinner
> in honor of
> The Surgeon General of the United States
> on Saturday, the fifteenth of July
> at eight o'clock
> The Naval Officers' Club
> Bethesda, Maryland
>
> RSVP   Reception, 7:00 PM
> (301) 555-4000   Service Dress Blue

Order of Precedence

In official interactions and at ceremonial and social occasions, deferential respect may be given to the position that an individual holds. Such positions are prioritized according to society's perception of the importance of that office.

Protocol governs the precedence given to positions in government, ecclesiastical and diplomatic life. In the U.S. government, such official positions are attained through election or appointment to an office, or by promotion within a uniformed service.

Official positions in the government are assigned relative levels of importance, with the President holding the highest level of precedence. The official precedence lists do not cover all positions, in which case precedence is determined by consideration of an individual's prominence within their organization and career field.

Diplomatic precedence is set by international agreement dating from the Congress of Vienna in 1815, and includes other criteria such as the date that diplomats present their credentials.

The military is very evident in the application of precedence according to grade. By custom, uniformed service officers of the same grade are ranked by date of rank; if the dates of rank are the same, then by total active service date and, if the same, officers in the Regular Corps take precedence among themselves according to their position on the permanent promotion list. Active duty officers precede Reserve officers, and Reserve officers precede retired officers of the same rank. In a ceremonial or social setting, a spouse is generally accorded the same ranking as the principal to whom precedence is given.

In the PHS, considerations of precedence are usually limited to an individual's military rank. Officers should nonetheless be cognizant of this social code, particularly when high ranking, nonmilitary officials are in attendance at official functions.

Receiving Line

A receiving line is used to afford those in attendance an opportunity to meet and greet the host and honored guest. It is typically held for about 30 minutes, and up to 45 minutes in duration for large receptions.

The receiving line should be in a location that does not disrupt guest flow to the reception area. A table may be placed behind the official party in the receiving line for water. Flags are arranged behind the table in order of precedence: the U.S. flag at the position of honor (i.e., the flag's own right), followed by Departmental or organizational flag, and then an admiral's flag. There are no firm rules for the formation of receiving lines, other than the host and honored guest position themselves at the head of the line, with spouses on their left, and all other officers are arrayed to the left in single file in order of rank. For official receptions, the customary order is a follows:

[Aide] ~ Host ~ Host's Spouse ~ Guest of Honor ~ Honored Guest's Spouse

or

[Aide] ~ Host ~ Guest of Honor ~ Honored Guest's Spouse ~ Host's Spouse

When the guest of honor is a head of state, the line is rearranged as follows:

[Aide] ~ Guest of Honor ~ Honored Guest's Spouse ~ Host ~ Host's Spouse

An announcer may be at the head of the receiving line to receive the names of each guest/couple in the waiting line. The announcer normally is an aide or other officer. The announcer introduces the guest to the host who, in turn, presents the guest to the guest of honor. Sometimes a "set-up" aide will be stationed several feet before the receiving line to give directions to those waiting in line. At large receptions, an officer may be positioned just off the end of the receiving line to direct guests to the main reception area.

Guests in the waiting line arrange themselves in either of two ways: women precede men, as is traditional; or, officers/officials precede their spouses or guests—the latter arrangement is customary at official functions of the Air Force, Navy, and Marine Corps.

In either case, the officer uses his/her official title and name ("Captain Alice Carter and Mr. Carter"). If an aide is receiving names, guests do not greet or shake hands with the aide. Guests should avoid starting a conversation with the host or guest of honor but, if so, keep it brief. In proceeding down a lengthy receiving line, guests should simply offer their name, shake hands and greet each person in the receiving line. Guests should never be holding a drink or food while meeting the official party in a receiving line.

Seating Arrangements

There are several seating arrangements that depend on the formality and type of occasion and the guest composition. Two representative arrangements are the mixed dinner table and head/speaker's table. If a mixed dinner is held (Figure 1.), the host and hostess sit at the head and foot of the table. When the occasion is a large official dinner with long tables, the host and hostess move to the center of the lengthwise sides of the table.

All other guests are seated according to their rank. The senior ranking/honored male guest is seated at the right of the hostess, and the senior ranking/honored female guest is at the right of the host. The second ranking man sits to the left of the hostess and the second ranking female sits to the host's left, and so on thereafter.

HOST				
	Ranking			
1	Woman	Woman	2	
3	Man	Man	4	
4	Woman	Woman	3	
2	Man	Man	1	
HOSTESS				

Figure 1. Mixed Table

←
3rd Rank Guest
Honored Guest
HOST/CHAIR
2nd Rank Guest
Toastmaster
Guest

Figure 2. Head/Speakers Table

Note that a spouse is accorded the same rank as the principal (i.e., the person in whom rank is vested). Thus, when a senior ranking man is seated to the right of the hostess, his wife will normally be seated to the right of the host if no senior ranking/honored female guest displaces her. If the spouse is also an officer or holds an official position with precedence ranking, that person is seated in accordance with his/her rank.

Whereas the place of honor is always to the right of the host/hostess, that position conveys to a senior ranking guest according to the rules of precedence. In order to allow an honored guest to be seated in the place of honor when a higher-ranking person is present, the host may want to ask the ranking guest to waive his seating right, if appropriate, or make the ranking guest a co-host of the event.

The seating protocol should be followed for formal dinners; however, officers will likely sit with their spouses at most occasions that are sponsored by the PHS and related organizations. For some occasions such as parties and retirements, spouses should be seated side-by-side. In these instances, the wife sits to the right of the husband, who assists with the wife's chair.

When being seated, diners should move to the right of the chair and sit from their left side. This will lessen the possibility of chairs or people bumping into one another.

Toasts

Toasting originated in the sixteenth century with the English custom of adding a small piece of spiced toast to flavor wine, and the term came to be applied to a drink proposed in honor of a person. A toast to honor individuals or institutions lends special significance to an event. All guests should participate, allowing the host, a senior officer or the official who organized a dinner to make the first toast. This is typically done once the dessert is served and the wine or champagne glasses are filled (never use liqueur or a mixed drink). Nonalcoholic beverage drinkers may raise their empty or filled wine glass (if filled, they need not drink from it), or sip from a water-filled glass during the toast (note, however, that in some military messes it is considered highly improper to drink a toast with water). Water only is used by all participants for toasts that honor those who are missing in action or prisoners of war.

A toast should be relatively brief, relevant to the individual and always on a warm and laudatory note; an injection of humor may impart a "lift" to the toast, as well (note that formal and diplomatic toasts to an individual are made to that person's official position). The person making the toast should stand and project in a clear voice while raising his/her glass in a salute. At formal occasions, the toastmaster stands to propose the toast, and guests rise before or after to respond to the toast; non-active duty women can remain seated unless the host's wife rises. For less formal occasions, all guests can remain seated. At the conclusion of the toast, guests should turn and, looking at the person who was toasted, raise their glass; the person's name may be repeated in unison and a sip of wine is then taken.

The person who is honored remains seated and does not drink to the toast, but should nod in acknowledgment. After the toast, he/she may rise to offer a toast with words of thanks.

Planning

Planning for a formal reception begin two to three months in advance of the event date. For those officers tasked with planning a reception, a planning checklist is provided in Appendix B.

Presentation of Awards

Awards/decoration ceremonies are held when a number of officers are to be recipients. The presentation of awards in a formal ceremony enhances the significance of the achievements being recognized and serves to bolster esprit de corps among the ranks. The presenting officer should be superior in rank or position to the highest ranking officer being decorated. A master of ceremonies, hereinafter referred to as adjutant, will direct the program. While the awards ceremony is attended principally by PHS officers, a recipient's colleagues and family are welcome to attend.

Organizational Sponsor
The USPHS routinely sponsors a semi-annual or an annual awards ceremony in the Washington, DC metropolitan area. PHS awards are also presented at Federal agency awards ceremonies when those awards relate to specific agency programs that the recipient has worked on.

Those officers being recognized whose duty station is outside of OpDiv Headquarters (typically the Washington, DC metropolitan area) are often more appropriately honored at ceremonies hosted by local organizational units to allow attendance by colleagues, family and friends.

Event Formality
The formality of the awards ceremony will vary consistent with the organizational level of the host unit, the rank of presiding officials and dignitaries, the location, number of officers being recognized, and resources. Within the Washington, DC area, when the Surgeon General or other similarly high-ranking officer is officiating, the awards ceremony is relatively formal and may include the PHS Honor Corps and Music Ensemble.

General Format
A typical awards ceremony program might appear as follows:

Sample Program Pamphlet

— Program —

Arrival Honors
Presentation of the Colors
  Surgeon General's Honor Corps
The National Anthem
  PHS Music Ensemble
Welcome
  RADM Kenneth Moritsugu
  Master of Ceremony
Opening Remarks
  VADM Richard H. Carmona
  United States Surgeon General
Presentations
The PHS March
  PHS Music Ensemble
Closing Remarks
Closing Honors
Reception

U.S. Public Health Service Commissioned Corps The *U.S. Surgeon General's* AWARDS CEREMONY July 22, 2008 1330 Lister Hill Auditorium, NIH Bethesda, MD	*Program* [See above]	*Awards* [List awards by precedence; start with highest] ***Distinguished Service Medal*** [List officers by rank, first name, last name, and office/agency] ***SG Medallion*** *Etc.*	*Ceremony Work Group* [Persons who assist with preparations] *Members of the SG Honor Corps Music Ensemble* *USPHS March* [Provide verses]
Pamphlet Cover	**Inside Pages**	**Inside Pages**	**Back Page**

Arrival. The adjutant begins by requesting guests to "please rise for the arrival of the official party" and calling the room to attention, at which time senior officials enter and proceed to the staging area.

Opening. The event opens with presentation of the colors and the national anthem. The adjutant then invites the audience to be seated; he/she welcomes the attendees and introduces officials at the front of the room. Opening remarks are made by the senior officer and/or agency official.

Award Presentations. Awards are presented in order of precedence, from highest to lowest. The adjutant announces "Attention to Orders," in response to which all officers stand at attention and others in the audience rise. The award citation is read for the first awards. The audience is invited to be seated. The adjutant calls one officer at a time, or a group of officers receiving a particular award, to the stage. The officer being recognized takes a position of attention to the left of the senior officer. A group of officers form a line to the left of the senior officer, facing the audience. The adjutant or senior officer may make remarks about the officer/group being recognized, and the senior officer attaches the award to the officer's uniform. If a large group, the senior officer attaches the award to one officer's uniform while an aide hands each of the other officers the written citation with award.

The senior officer shakes the hand of the recognized officer, who then salutes the senior officer. The adjutant initiates applause, and the award recipient exits the staging area.

The program cycle is repeated for each type of award.

Closing. The senior officer/official makes closing remarks. At the conclusion of those remarks, the adjutant asks the audience to rise while the official party departs. Once the official party has left, the adjutant announces "This concludes the awards ceremony. Please join the award recipients for a reception in the (location)."

Sample Staging Area

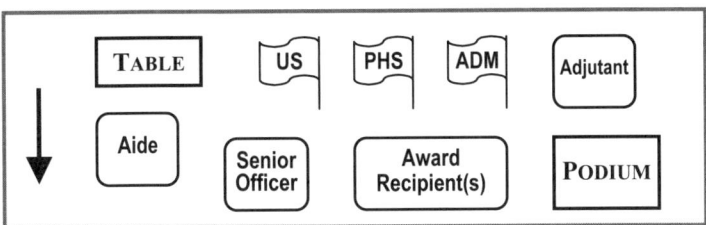

Planning

Planning and preparations for a formal awards ceremony should begin about three months in advance of the event date. Less formal occasions may be planned with much less advance time, in accordance with the ceremony particulars. For those officers tasked with planning an awards ceremony, a planning checklist is provided in Appendix C.

Promotion Ceremony

Uniformed services traditionally hold promotion ceremonies to formally acknowledge and publicly recognize an officer's appointment to a higher rank. The achievement of a promotion is a significant event in the life of an officer, and the presence of fellow officers serves to reinforce esprit de corps among the ranks. The presenting officer should be superior in rank or position to the highest ranking officer being promoted. A master of ceremonies, hereinafter referred to as adjutant, will direct the program. Family and friends are invited to share in the officer's achievement and participate in the ceremony.

Organizational Sponsor
Public Health Service officers work in several principal agencies of the Federal government that are hierarchically segmented into operating divisions (OpDivs), agencies, areas/bureaus/centers/institutes, and then service units or offices. Depending on the number of officers being promoted and the organizational units they represent, the promotion ceremony is hosted by the highest organizational level starting at the operating division or agency level.

Those officers being promoted whose duty station is outside of OpDiv headquarters (typically the Washington, DC metropolitan area) are, in most instances, more appropriately honored at ceremonies hosted by local organizational units to allow greater participation and attendance by colleagues, family and friends.

Event Formality
The formality of the promotion ceremony will vary consistent with the organizational level of the host unit, the rank of presiding officials and dignitaries, the location, number of officers being promoted, and resources. Within the Washington, D.C. area, when the Surgeon General or other high-ranking officer is officiating, the promotion ceremony is usually quite formal and may include the PHS Honor Corps and Music Ensemble.

Event Invitations
An invitation is sent to the promoted officer's family, with a request for a family member or close friend to participate in replacing the old shoulder boards with the new. Supervisors are invited, as are fellow officers and colleagues who may be sent a general invitation. The highest ranking official of the host organization and the highest ranking PHS commissioned officer in that area are invited, with the senior officer officiating if an Admiral. In addition, other high level officials within the organization should be invited.

Event Scheduling
Whereas officers are promoted on the first day of the quarter in which they are eligible, the majority receive their promotions effective 1 July. For that

reason, most organizational units schedule one promotion ceremony to cover the entire year and invite all officers who are to be promoted during that year to be recognized at the ceremony.

General Format
A typical promotion ceremony program might appear as follows:

**Sample
Program
Pamphlet**

— *Program* —

Arrival Honors
Presentation of the Colors
Surgeon General's Honor Corps
The National Anthem
PHS Music Ensemble
Welcome
RADM Mary Smith
NIH Commissioned Corps Liaison Officer
Opening Remarks
William Kennedy, Ph.D.
Director, National Institutes of Health
Promotion
William Kennedy, Ph.D.
ADM Mary Smith
CAPT David Everett, Adjutant
The PHS March
PHS Music Ensemble
Closing Remarks
Closing Honors
Reception

The Tenth Annual National Institutes of Health **PROMOTION CEREMONY** for **U.S. Public Health Service Commissioned Officers** July 15, 2008 1330 Natcher Auditorium, NIH Bethesda, MD	*Program* [See above]	*Promotions* *To Captain:* [List officers by last name, first name, category and, if applicable, agency/institute] *To Commander:* Etc.	*NIH* [Agencies/Institutes] *Ceremony Work Group* [Persons who assist with preparations] Members of the SG Honor Corps Music Ensemble *USPHS March* [Provide verses] Special thanks to family, colleagues
Pamphlet Cover	**Inside Pages**	**Inside Pages**	**Back Page**

Arrival. The adjutant begins by requesting guests to "please rise for the arrival of the official party" and calling the room to attention, at which time senior officials enter and proceed to the staging area.

Opening. The event opens with presentation of the colors and the national anthem. The adjutant then invites the audience to be seated; he/she welcomes the attendees and introduces officials at the front of the room. Opening remarks are made by the senior officer and/or agency official.

Promotions. Promotion is by order of rank, from highest to lowest. The adjutant announces "Attention to Orders," in response to which all officers stand at attention and others in the audience rise. The promotion order is read for the first promotion rank. The audience is invited to be seated. The adjutant calls one officer at a time to the stage to be promoted; the officer and family member (or designee if no family member is present) proceed to the stage. The officer being promoted takes a position of attention to the left of the senior officer, and the family member stands to the left of the officer. The adjutant or senior officer may make remarks about the officer and/or introduce the family member who will assist in the promotion. The adjutant hands the correct shoulder boards to the senior officer and family member, who replace the old with the new shoulder boards.

The senior officer shakes the hand of the promoted officer, who then salutes the senior officer. The adjutant initiates applause, and the promoted officer and family member exit the stage.

The program cycle is repeated for each promotion rank.

Closing. The senior officer/official makes closing remarks. At the conclusion of those remarks, the adjutant asks the audience to rise while the official party departs. Once the official party has left, the adjutant announces "This concludes the promotion ceremony. Please join us for a reception in the (location)."

Sample Staging Area

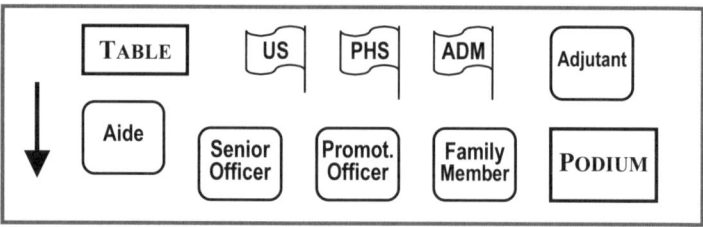

Planning

Planning and preparations for a formal promotion ceremony should begin three to four months in advance of the event date. Less formal occasions may be planned with much less advance time, in accordance with the ceremony particulars. For those officers tasked with planning a promotion ceremony, a planning checklist is provided in Appendix C.

Retirement Ceremony

It is a tradition within uniformed services to hold retirement ceremonies to formally acknowledge and publicly recognize an officer's honorable service. This is an important occasion for all officers—the retiree and the active duty officers in attendance—and warrants the attention of senior officials to ensure a proper send-off. The retiring officer should be leaving the service with an expression of appreciation for his/her valued work over the years, and with the knowledge that he will continue to be looked upon as a member of the PHS family in retirement. A master of ceremonies, hereinafter referred to as the presiding officer, will direct the program. This person may be a senior official or an officer colleague of the retiree.

Event Formality
The formality of the retirement ceremony will vary consistent with the rank of the retiring officer, the rank of presiding officials and dignitaries, and whether more than one officer is being retired. When the Surgeon General or other similarly high-ranking officer is officiating, the ceremony may be quite formal and include the PHS Honor Corps and Music Ensemble.

It is appropriate at a retirement ceremony to present the officer with recognition of his career contributions to the Corps (e.g., the PHS Citation). It is also a nice gesture to prepare a presentation case holding the national flag and devices (e.g., medals and ribbons) that were earned by the retiring officer. In the PHS, the retirement ceremony is a farewell event at which fellow officers, colleagues, family and friends are present, and gifts are presented to the retiree (cf., a formal military ceremony where gifts and mementos may be withheld during the ceremony).

Event Preparations
The selection of an event location and other particulars, such as the guest speakers and invited guests, should be discussed with the retiring officer. If high-ranking officials are among the official party, planners need to contact those persons regarding their availability before deciding on a date for the ceremony.

The sending of formal invitations should be considered. Usually, a general invitation is sent by a broadcast e-mail to fellow officers and colleagues within the officer's duty station, and to others specified by the retiring officer, with a request for response. The retiring officer's family and close friends are invited by personal communication, and supervisors and senior officials in the retiree's duty station should be invited individually.

Certain items need to be planned well in advance of the ceremony. For example, a determination of the ceremony location, date, and official party, to include the presiding officer and guest speakers, needs to be set. If an award is planned, there typically is an extended lead time necessary for approval and transmittal. If a national flag that is flown over a specified site (e.g., U.S. Capitol building) and/or a letter of recognition from an elected official are desired, those items need attention early in the ceremony preparations.

General Format

The program formality and content can vary considerably. When accompanied by a meal, the ceremony should commence after the meal is finished. A typical retirement ceremony program may include the following:

Sample Program Pamphlet

— *Program* —

Arrival Honors
Presentation of the Colors
Surgeon General's Honor Corps
The National Anthem
PHS Music Ensemble
Invocation
Welcome and Opening Remarks
RADM Mary Smith
Director, National Cancer Institute
Guest Speakers
[Names and Positions]
Presentation of Awards, Gifts, Tributes
**Reading of Retirement Orders and
    Presentation of Retirement Certificate**
Presentation to Mrs. Franklin
Musical Selection
PHS Music Ensemble
Honoree's Remarks
The PHS March
PHS Music Ensemble
Closing Honors
Reception

(Continued on next page.)

Sample Program Pamphlet

U.S. Public Health Service Commissioned Corps Retirement Ceremony to Honor CAPT Benjamin Franklin November 29, 2007 1300 Park Building Rockville, MD	[Biosketch of retiring officer, to include academic degrees, positions held, accomplishments]	*Program* [See above]	*Special Thanks* [List of persons who assist with preparations] Members of the SG Honor Corps Music Ensemble *USPHS March* [Provide verses] Many thanks to family, colleagues and friends
Pamphlet Cover	**Inside, Page 2**	**Inside, Page 3**	**Back Page**

Arrival. For a formal event, the official party is escorted as a group to their seats. Family members usually take seats in the first row of the audience, followed by the presiding officer, senior officer, retiree and other ceremony participants who sit in front, and facing the audience (spouse may elect to sit with the retiree).

Opening. The event may open with presentation of the colors, the national anthem (other musical selections may be performed during the ceremony) and an invocation. The presiding officer begins with opening remarks and introductions of those at the front of the room.

Guest Speakers. The guest speakers will address the audience, with the presiding officer or principal speaker assigned the task of summarizing the retiring officer's career and contributions to the PHS.

Presentations. When the program calls for presentation of a decoration, the presiding officer so announces and the retiring officer takes a position of attention to the left of the senior officer. The senior officer will read the citation, attach the decoration to the retiring officer's uniform and present the written citation to the retiring officer. The senior officer shakes the hand of the retiring officer, who then salutes the senior officer (if superior in rank to the retiring officer). Gifts, to include the presentation case, are presented to the retiree at this time. Personal tributes to the retiree may also be made at this time.

Retirement Orders. The presiding officer will announce "Attention to Orders," in response to which all officers stand at attention and others in the audience rise for the reading of the retirement order. The retiring officer rises and takes a position next to the senior officer. After the order is read, the senior officer presents the *Retirement Certificate* to the retiree.

Recognitions. The presiding officer will then invite the audience to be seated, and the retiree's family or other significant individuals are invited to come forward for recognition—a *Certificate of Appreciation* and/or flowers may be presented to the retiree's spouse.

Honoree's Remarks and Closing Honors. The retiree is invited to make farewell remarks. At the conclusion of those remarks, the presiding officer asks the audience to rise while the official party, led by the retiree and spouse, depart. Because the USPHS traces its origins to ministering to merchant seamen, the retired officer may be piped with the Navy custom of sounding gongs or bells to announce a senior officer's arrival or departure from a ship. In the PHS retirement ceremony, this symbolizes the retired officer leaving a ship and going ashore for the last time.

The presiding officer announces:

"As CAPT Franklin completes his career with the Public Health Service and retires as a commissioned officer with 30 years of active service to his Country, we ring four bells to signify his departure."

The retiring officer, facing the presiding officer, requests departure:

"Sir, as I have been properly relieved, request permission to leave the deck and to retire." Presiding officer responds: "Permission granted."

The presiding officer announces: "Sound (2, 4, 6, or 8) bells, (rank and retiree's name), departing."

Note that a ship's bell is rung in pairs—a set of two rings in quick succession are equivalent to one bell, which is followed by a brief interlude before the next bell. The appropriate number of bells for each pay grade is as follows:

Officers in grades 0-4 and below:	*2 Bells*
Officers in grades 0-5 and 0-6:	*4 Bells*
Officers in grades 0-7 and 0-8:	*6 Bells*
Officers in grades 0-9 and above:	*8 Bells*

Program planners may want to include two facing ranks (columns) of not more than eight officers, through which the retired officer walks as the bell is rung.

Reception. Once the official party has left, an assisting officer announces "Ladies and gentlemen, this concludes the ceremony. Please join (name of retiree) for a reception and ceremonial cutting of the cake in the (location)." The retired officer returns to cut the first pieces of cake with a PHS sword, and then stands in an area away from the cake to receive and greet guests.

Sample Staging Area

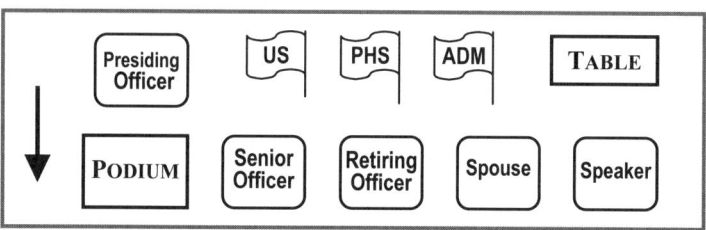

Planning

Planning and preparations for a formal retirement ceremony should begin at least three months in advance of the event date, keeping in mind the items previously discussed that may need additional lead time. Less formal occasions may be planned with less advance time, in accordance with the ceremony particulars. For those officers tasked with planning a retirement ceremony, a planning checklist is provided in Appendix C.

SECTION IV.
SPECIAL DUTY

The USPHS offers opportunities to serve the Commissioned Corps in ways that will enrich an officer's career experience. Officers should consider becoming involved in special duty assignments, which can be personally fulfilling and also build camaraderie and esprit de corps within the Corps.

AIDE-DE-CAMP
BOARDS
CHIEF PROFESSIONAL OFFICER
ESCORT OFFICER
HONOR CORPS
JUNIOR OFFICER ADVISORY GROUP
LIAISON, COMMISSIONED CORPS
MINORITY OFFICERS LIAISON COUNCIL
MUSIC ENSEMBLE
PROFESSIONAL ADVISORY COMMITTEE
PROTOCOL OFFICER
READINESS FORCE
RECRUITER
SURGEON GENERAL'S POLICY ADVISORY COUNCIL

Aide-de-Camp

The aide-de-camp (French: *camp assistant*) is an officer who acts in the capacity of a fulltime confidential assistant to a flag officer—one who carries the rank of Admiral or General at grade O-7 and above. The role of military aide was adopted from the European tradition during the American Revolution, beginning with those who served as aides to General George Washington. Aides are often selected for their leadership abilities, and they have played a significant part in American military history. It is a mark of distinction to serve as an aide, and it presents a rare opportunity to observe senior officers in positions of leadership. It is well known that a substantial proportion of aides go on to become military leaders in their own right.

The aide-de-camp (ADC) provides administrative support and performs a range of assistive duties. The aide is called upon to provide assistance and serve as a ready resource to relieve high-ranking civilian and uniformed service officials (hereinafter referred to as "the principal") of everyday matters. The Surgeon General, Deputy Surgeon General and other flag officers and government dignitaries may have the services of an aide.

Qualifications
Those who serve as an aide should have certain basic qualifications. The ADC must first meet all professional, medical and fitness standards.
Knowledge. The PHS aide needs to be knowledgeable about military custom, courtesy, protocol and social etiquette. It is important that the aide have a good understanding of the U.S. Public Health Service—its history, mission, organization and operational policies, and familiarity with the agencies to which PHS officers are assigned.
Personal Qualities. An aide must be self-reliant and resourceful. He/she is able to organize, prioritize and carry out assigned duties competently with little or no guidance—this should not preclude the aide from asking when uncertain. He is skilled in both verbal and written communications, and adept at dealing appropriately with people at all organizational levels. The ability to make sound judgments in the absence of specific instruction is vital.

The ADC must have an exemplary military appearance and bearing. Because his actions reflect directly upon the principal who chose him, it is imperative that the aide conduct both his official duties and personal life responsibly. The aide must have integrity and convey professionalism in order to earn the respect of the principal and others with whom the aide interacts. And, the aide is expected to be circumspect with regard to anything said or done by the principal that is not meant to be publicly divulged.

Carrying Out Responsibilities
The ADC must subordinate his own desires to the needs of the principal. In this regard, the aide should take time to become acquainted with the principal's work habits, interests and preferences. In that way, he will achieve the principal's confidence and trust in his ability to make appropriate decisions.

The aide understands that fraternization with the principal is not allowed when the public and subordinates are present. The ADC is not to alter the requirement for a professional manner and adherence to military protocol while in public view. He should also be mindful that his official relationship with the principal does not confer command status. His demeanor must always conform to that which is expected of a subordinate, and show the proper respect accorded to ranking officers.

Duties

The aide-de-camp is responsible for a multitude of tasks, some of which may be shared with other personnel such as the principal's secretarial and support staff. The scope of the aide's duties will also vary depending on the needs of the principal to whom assigned. The aide is responsible for administrative matters that may include scheduling, monitoring appointments, handling correspondence, carrying messages on behalf of the principal, vetting requests for the principal's time, serving at the start of a receiving line to introduce guests to the principal, and advising the principal on rules of protocol and etiquette. The aide will also be responsible for planning and coordinating the principal's participation at official ceremonies and meetings, and for briefing the principal on all relevant matters that pertain to such participation.

An aide assists the principal in meeting the demands of a work schedule, by facilitating the movement of the principal throughout the day. This may include, for example, accompanying the principal at various meetings, meeting people and making proper introductions. The ADC should always maintain a low profile and stay at a distance from the principal, but remain near enough to support the principal when needed.

The aide has significant responsibilities that relate to official travel by the principal. Travel preparations—developing the itinerary, making contacts with the host organization, and numerous other tasks need to be accomplished with skill and competency. Upon return, the aide may be charged with preparing reimbursement vouchers, trip reports and thank you notes, as appropriate. See the Section, *Escort Officer,* for more detailed information regarding the aide's responsibilities when accompanying the principal on official business that involves travel.

Dress and Grooming

An aide's dress and grooming should be impeccable. His wardrobe, which may be necessarily extensive, is maintained in conformance with all uniform standards. A secure knowledge of the proper dress for different occasions is essential, both for himself and when he may be called upon to advise the principal. The ADC must always have a bag packed and be prepared for any occasion that requires the appropriate uniform. It is also advised that the ADC have a uniform at the office, along with extra accoutrements in the rare case the principal may lack an item.

The PHS aide's uniform is distinguished by the wearing of an aiguillette on the left shoulder. The number of cords that comprise the aiguillette signify the rank of the principal, as follows: two cords, RADM; three cords, VADM; and four cords, 4-star ADM and those deemed equivalent or above (e.g., Secretary, Assistant/Under Secretary of DHHS). The aiguillette signifies the position of the wearer and provides an assurance of cooperation by others. The aide should always be well groomed, keeping in mind the following: hair is clean, trimmed and neatly styled; jewelry is minimal; personal articles such as pens and combs are kept so not to be visible; and, ensure good oral hygiene, and use cologne/perfume sparingly.

Boards

The USPHS administers several boards that provide program support for the Office of Commissioned Corps Operations. PHS officers who meet specified criteria may volunteer to serve on a board, which provides an interesting and worthwhile experience for the officer and a valuable service to the Corps. Among the more prominent boards are the following:
- Appointment Board (AB)—Appointment Boards assess the fitness and qualifications of candidates for appointment to the Regular and Reserve Corps. ABs are comprised of three or more active duty officers, the majority of whom are in the same professional category as the candidates for which the board is convened. To be considered for this board, an officer must be in the Regular Corps, be at the senior grade (0-5) and above and have at least five years of PHS Commissioned Corps active duty experience. Officers are appointed to serve for one year.
- Medical Review Board (MRB)—Medical Review Boards review the cases of officers whose physical examination (PE) results might indicate possible disqualification for further service, officers who are on temporary disability and are required to undergo periodic PE, and officers who may be entitled to retirement due to physical disability. The MRBs are comprised of three senior grade officers (0-5) and above, at least one of whom shall be a medical officer. For the Medical Appeals Board, three or more medical officers are required.
- Promotion Boards—The Annual Temporary Promotion Board (ATPB) and Annual Permanent Promotion Board (APPB) assess the fitness and qualifications of Regular and Reserve Corps officers for temporary and permanent promotion, respectively, to the next higher grade. One or more ATPBs/APPBs are constituted at least once in a calendar year for each professional category. ATPBs/APPBs are comprised of three or more officers at the rank/grade of Director (0-6), the majority of whom must be in the Regular Corps and in the same professional category (insofar as it is practicable) as the officers to be examined for promotion. No officer may serve as a member of either board for the same category or group more frequently than once every three years. An effort is made to ensure that the ATPB/APPB membership is representative with respect to agency/OpDiv and field representation.

Service on these and other boards generally require that board members maintain in confidence all information with respect to individual officers and the proceedings.

Chief Professional Officer

A Chief Professional Officer (CPO) is the official representative of his/her respective commissioned officer professional category. CPOs provide leadership and direction for the category, and serve as the advocate for the category in areas of interest to the Corps. In addition, a CPO is the liaison between the professional category and the Office of the Surgeon General.

The selection of a CPO in the dental, engineer, nurse, and pharmacist categories is required by statute, and includes promotion of the nominee to a temporary flag grade for the duration of service as a CPO.

The Surgeon General may also appoint a CPO for other professional categories when it would benefit the PHS; however, there is no requirement for promotion of these nominees to a flag grade. It has been customary to appoint a CPO for all professional categories.

Eligibility

To be considered for the position of a CPO, an officer must meet certain eligibility criteria. These generally include the following.

- Be appointed in, and hold his PHS commission as a member of, the professional category for which the CPO is to be selected.
- Be a member of the Regular Corps and hold either the temporary or permanent pay grade of O-6.
- Have served at least 12 years of active duty with the uniformed services. At least six years on active duty must be as a PHS officer. Must meet the basic level of force readiness standards.
- Have no more than 30 years of service creditable for purposes of determining retirement eligibility at the time of nomination.
- Maintain current professional licensure when required, and meet any additional category-specific criteria.

Because the CPO appointment is in addition to the responsibilities an individual has in his permanent duty assignment, a prospective nominee's agency must agree to the nominee serving up to a four-year term, and it has the option to approve or deny any extension beyond the nominee's mandatory retirement date.

Personal and Professional Qualities

The CPO should be a person of integrity, with demonstrated leadership and management abilities. The CPO will serve as a distinguished role model to all officers in the CPO's professional category, so the prospective candidate needs to be highly regarded among his peers and others with whom that person is known. A CPO Nomination Board is convened for each professional category to evaluate the professional credentials of candidates. Principal criteria include the following.

- Annual performance ratings on the Commissioned Officers' Effectiveness Reports.
- Awards received from the PHS and other uniformed services.
- Education, licensure status, and any special professional qualifications.
- Scope and variety of assignments and responsibilities over the course of the individual's career.
- Recommendations from current and past agency heads and other senior officials.

Following its review of all eligible candidates, the CPO Nomination Board will select no more than five officers who will be rated as either qualified or highly qualified. The Board's recommendations will be forwarded to the Surgeon General for final decision.

CPOs are appointed for a period of four years. Any CPO continuing to serve past four years does so in the capacity of Acting CPO. Individuals appointed may be removed at any time as the Surgeon General may direct.

Escort Officer

An escort officer refers to the officer who is temporarily assigned to a flag officer or dignitary ("the principal"). A *local* escort officer may be assigned to meet and accompany the principal (also referred to as a distinguished visitor or DV) who is arriving from out-of-town. The escort will brief the principal and guide that person in accordance with the official itinerary.

The aide-de-camp (see the Section, *Aide-de-Camp*) and escort officer perform duties that are quite similar when the principal is on official business. An escort officer typically does not wear an aide's aiguillette; however, in the PHS, escort officers may be accorded this custom in recognition of their responsibility, and to make others aware that an official duty is being performed. In both roles—aide-de-camp and escort officer—PHS officers are called upon to provide information and assistance in support of the principal.

A *protocol officer* refers to an officer or civilian who provides fulltime management and support service to commanders with respect to visits by distinguished visitors, travel, conferences, recognition programs, special ceremonies and social functions. The protocol officer also advises the commander and staff on military customs and courtesies, history, organization and policy. Escort officers will be coordinating a principal's visit with the protocol officer when one is present. See the Section, *Protocol Officer,* for detailed information.

Personal Qualities

Like an aide-de-camp, the escort officer must have an exemplary military appearance and bearing. He/she should be familiar with military customs, courtesies, protocol and social etiquette. He must be self-reliant, resourceful, and able to organize and carry out a myriad of tasks competently and with good judgment. His grooming and uniforms are maintained in accordance with the highest standards.

Distinguished Visitor

A distinguished visitor may be a high-ranking PHS officer such as the Surgeon General, a civilian official of the Department of Health and Human Services (HHS), or any individual or group identified in the Department of Defense *Table of Precedence*. A visit by a DV is an important event and it is essential that thorough planning and preparation be accomplished for the visit to be a success.

Escort Basics

The DV travels to conduct official business, and it is important that the logistical side of the visit be accomplished efficiently and competently. The escort should keep the following in mind.

- Always be well groomed, and wear a clean and pressed uniform.
- Always be on time and earlier if possible.
- Always practice military courtesy and adhere to official protocol.
- Always act professionally and maintain a formal military bearing while in public view.
- Always remember that you must subordinate your desires to the needs of the DV.

Notification

Upon receiving notification, the local escort officer (hereinafter referred to as "escort") will ensure that information pertaining to the visit is received well in advance. The escort should call the DV's office and, if the DV is the Surgeon General or Deputy Surgeon General, also call the aide. The escort should introduce himself, request information about the visit and provide contact information. Pertinent information includes the following.

- Purpose and dates of visit.
- Names and titles of those in the official party, and a picture(s) if necessary.
- Itinerary, including a detailed schedule of daily activities and locations of same.
- Travel information, including mode of transportation, arrival and departure times, and ground transportation requirements.
- Accommodations information, including pre-existing or needed reservations.

- Special needs or requests, such as dietary restrictions, entertainment, rest periods.
- When the DV's spouse is also traveling, information about the spouse's participation and need for social activities during the DV's official visit.

Pre-Arrival Preparations
The escort will ensure that the following arrangements have been made prior to arrival of the DV.
Arrival and Ground Transportation
- Ensure that a full sized vehicle (if available) is reserved and the driver, whether the escort or another person, knows the directions and actual route to the DV's destinations.
- Unless waived by the DV, arrange for the senior officer or official to be present at the arrival and departure of a flag rank or equivalent civilian official.

Accommodations
- Ensure that lodging is appropriate and reserved.
- If the DV has an aide or escort traveling with him/her, ensure that their quarters are in keeping with their standing as a member of the official party.

Event Site and Itinerary
- Visit the location of event sites with the local coordinator in advance to learn details about the following: where the official car will stop and where it will be parked; who will greet the DV; the location of the facility entrance/exit; and, seating and stage arrangement. Review the written introduction and schedule of activities for the DV, and include an appropriate amount of time for the DV to personally greet people. Ensure that all arrangements conform to official protocol. Prepare written notes that can be given to the DV.
- Ensure that the itinerary provides sufficient time for occasional rest periods, coffee breaks, meals, change of clothes, and transportation. Review menu items to ensure they conform to any dietary restrictions.
- Confirm the dress requirement for all scheduled activities.
- Know about the availability of local dry cleaners, pharmacies, and emergency medical care.

Verification
- Call the DV's office and aide with any revisions to the itinerary and other information that may impact the DV's visit. If an event program is available, send it to the DV before the visit commences. Once verified, prepare other local officers to be on station ready status should they be needed.

DV's Arrival
The escort should follow certain steps to ensure a smooth DV pick-up.
Arrive Early
- Be present at the airport terminal or train depot arrival point about 30 minutes before the DV's scheduled arrival time. Coordinate with terminal security to position the car near the arrival point.
- Confirm the arrival time on visual displays inside the terminal and stand at the arrival gate (if security permits) to wait for the DV.

Meet DV
- Greet and introduce yourself to the DV—"Good morning (afternoon, evening), Admiral. I am (rank, first and last name) and I will be your escort officer during your visit."
- Assist with the DV's luggage.
- Open and close the car's right rear door for the DV, who will sit on the right side of the rear seat. If not driving, the escort either: (1) enters through the left rear door, safety permitting; or (2) enters the right rear door before the DV and slides across to the left side rear seat.
- Give a brief description of the day's itinerary. Provide the DV with a brief that includes the program, itinerary, notes, names of event principals, small map of the area, and your contact information.
- Carry all materials (e.g., brief case) for the DV throughout the visit.

From this moment forward, the escort officer is on duty until released by the DV.

Itinerary
If stopping at the lodging first, assist with luggage and accompany the DV to the hotel registration area. Once registered, agree on a time to meet in the lobby to proceed to the next destination or event. Inspect the DV's uniform in a private area before proceeding with the itinerary.

Plan to arrive at the scheduled event about 30 minutes beforehand and, upon arrival, escort the DV to the DV greeter. When walking with the DV, stay to that person's left and one-half pace behind. When approaching a door, the escort moves forward to hold the door open.

The escort will either assist the DV during the event or, if not directly involved, remain in the proximity of the DV. Keep easy eye contact with the DV and be prepared to assist, as needed.

The aide, escort and/or protocol officer may be responsible for numerous other tasks associated with a DV visit. PHS officers should consult protocol guidance documents for further information.

Planning
For those officers serving as an escort, a planning checklist is provided in Appendix D.

Honor Corps

The PHS Honor Corps was formed in 1999 by the Surgeon General and is known as "The Surgeon General's Own." The Honor Corps, also referred to as the PHS Honor Cadre, functions in the capacity of a military color guard. The military color guard derives from a time when flags were carried into battle, both as an identifying symbol and as a rallying point for troops. Today, that practice has been superseded by color guards who carry the colors (national and organizational flags) at military and civil ceremonies and events.

Mission
The Honor Corps represents the Office of the Surgeon General (OSG) by presenting the colors at ceremonial functions of the OSG, Public Health Service, HHS and non-HHS sponsored events.

Ceremonial Unit
The Ceremonial Unit presents the colors at appropriate ceremonies and events sponsored by the PHS, and agencies and operating divisions of HHS. Awards ceremonies, promotion ceremonies, retirement ceremonies, memorial services, and special events are among the types of venues served.

Basic Standards
The Honor Corps is composed of officers who have shown exceptional commitment to, and pride in the PHS Commissioned Corps. Honor Corps members must meet exceptionally high standards of professionalism to be selected for this special duty. To be considered, prospective members must be in excellent physical condition and meet certain height and weight standards and, without exception, have an exemplary military appearance and bearing.

Officers are considered probationary members for the first year of service in the Honor Corps. Inspection knowledge and precision drill are essential and this is accomplished through regularly scheduled practices. Officers should be thoroughly familiar with military courtesies, customs and protocol. Uniforms are worn daily with pride and distinction. Regular or permanent membership is granted when all uniforms deemed necessary for full participation are acquired; when the officer attains drill and ceremony proficiency; when attendance at practice and assigned ceremonial duties meets prescribed standards; and when the officer shows the ongoing positive attitude of an exemplary officer.

Color Guard
The U.S. flag is known as the national color or color *(singular)* and, when carried with organizational flags by color-bearing units, the flags together are referred to as colors. It is considered an honor for uniformed service personnel to carry the colors.

Composition

A color guard unit is normally comprised of four individuals: two color bearers in the center and one color guard on each side of the color bearers. Whereas in the armed forces each guard carries a rifle, in the PHS each guard carries a PHS sword. The national color is given the honor position on the marching right, with organizational and positional flags to the left. The senior officer in the color guard commands the unit.

Color Guard Formation

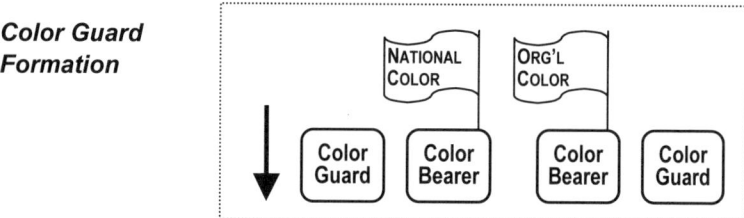

March

The color guard is formed and marched in one rank at close interval. The color guard marches at right shoulder arms, and wheels to the right or left to complete facing movements—these are executed with the command "Right (Left) Wheel, March." To complete a wheeling movement, the guard nearest the direction of turn serves as the pivot point by marching in place while turning in the new direction. The other members shorten their steps and turn together in an arc, keeping abreast of each other to maintain forward alignment. When the new direction is reached, each member marches in place until the command "Halt" or "Forward, March" is given.

Salutes

When passing in review, the senior officer commands "Eyes, Right" at the prescribed saluting distance and the organizational color salutes (dips), and resumes the carry at the command "Ready, Front." Note that the guard on the right flank does not execute Eyes Right, and that the national color renders no salute. The organizational color salutes in all military ceremonies while the national anthem, "To the Color," or a foreign national anthem is played, and when rendering honors to the organizational commander (PHS Surgeon General), his/her direct representative, or an officer of equivalent or higher grade.

Presentation of the Colors

Posting and retiring the colors refers to displaying the colors, placing the colors in flag stands, and taking away the colors. The following procedures are used for posting and retiring the colors indoors. In PHS ceremonies, the colors may be marched to the front of the room and placed in flag stands, or they may be retired immediately after the playing of the national anthem.

The color guard forms just outside the auditorium, dining or meeting room, and the audience is directed to stand for the colors and national anthem. The color guard enters in a line formation, preferably, or in a column and marches to the front center of the room, and then turns to face the audience. The unit's senior officer commands "Colors, Halt," and "Present, Arms," and reports to the host that "The Colors are present." The national anthem is played and, at its conclusion, the command is given to "Order, Arms." At this point, the color guard may either march to the flag stands or exit the room with the colors.

The figures below show five basic positions and movements associated with the sword when presenting the colors:

Figure 1. Position of attention.

Figure 2. Draw sword. Upon the command "Draw," grasp the scabbard with the left hand, turn it clockwise 180°, tilt it forward to form a 45° angle with the ground; take the sword grip in the right hand and pull it about 6 inches from the scabbard, with the right forearm parallel to the ground. On the command "Sword" the sword is pulled out of the scabbard and held in the position of Carry Sword.

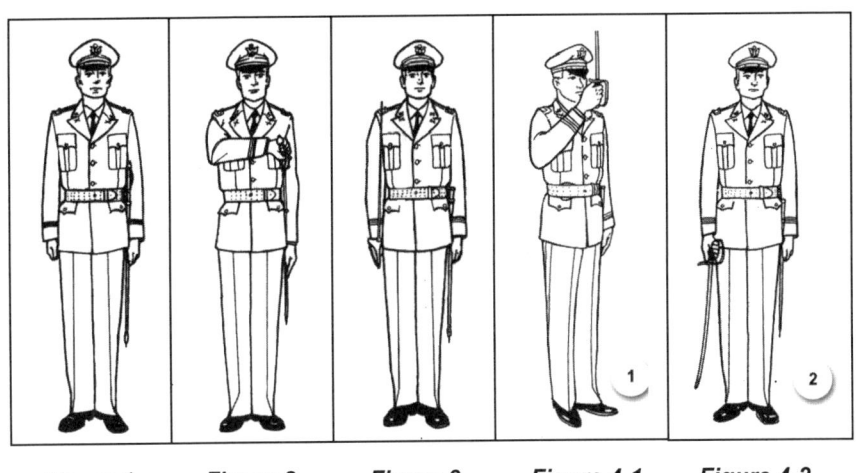

Figure 1   Figure 2   Figure 3   Figure 4-1   Figure 4-2

Source: U.S. Army Field Manual 3-21.5

Figure 3. Carry sword. The sword is held in the right hand, wrist straight as possible with the thumb along the seam of the trouser leg; the blade point rests inside the right shoulder.

Figure 4-1. Present sword. On the command "Present," the sword is brought to a position with the hilt to the chin, the flat of the blade about four inches from the nose, sword point up.

Figure 4-2. On the command "Arms" the right hand is lowered with the flat of the blade upward, the thumb extended on the left side of the grip, and the tip of the sword about 6 inches from the ground. On the command "Order, Arms" the sword is returned to the position of carry sword.

Junior Officer Advisory Group

The Junior Officer Advisory Group (JOAG) was officially chartered on December 7, 2001. It provides advice and consultation on interests and concerns specific to junior officers in the Commissioned Corps. Membership is for officers at the 0-1 to 0-4 grades, and an effort is made to have broad representation from among all PHS agencies staffed by junior officers. Junior officers are encouraged to actively participate in activities of the JOAG, because it is a good way to build fellowship and become more involved in the Commissioned Corps.

Mission
The Junior Officer Advisory Group provides advice and consultation to the Surgeon General, Professional Advisory Committees (PACs), Chief Professional Officers (CPOs), the Commissioned Officers Association and other Commissioned Corps groups on issues relating to professional practice and personnel activities that affect junior officers.

Objectives
The JOAG serves in a resource, advisory and liaison capacity to assist in the development and coordination of PHS professional activities related to junior officers with the following objectives:
- To identify and advocate on behalf of junior officer issues and concerns.
- To assist the Office of the Surgeon General, Office of Commissioned Corps Operations, the PACs and CPOs in the assessment of personnel needs, and in recruitment, training, utilization and recognition of junior officers.
- To develop position papers, statistical reports and/or guidelines where appropriate, to advise and comment on matters relating to personnel activities and professional practice affecting junior officers.
- To promote junior officer development and utilization.
- To promote cooperation and communication between junior and senior officers throughout the PHS.
- To serve as a liaison between junior officers and other PHS or external components, and provide advice and consultation to the agencies and operating divisions upon request.
- To serve as a communications link and information resource for junior officers.

Membership
Composition and Term. The Junior Officer Advisory Group is comprised of active duty members who are junior officers (temporary rank of 0-4 or below). The JOAG may have from 11 to 20 voting members; at least two of those members must be assigned to a duty station 75 or more miles from the Washington, DC metropolitan area. Efforts must be made to ensure that the

JOAG has broad representation from among all agencies, and does not consist entirely of one gender or race or ethnicity. Members serve a term of two years, not to exceed a cumulative total of four years.

Nomination. Voting member terms are staggered so that approximately one-half of the members' terms expire annually. The JOAG operational year begins October 1. Each year, the JOAG will solicit, through broadcast e-mail and newsletters, nominations (including self-nominations) for upcoming vacancies. The names of respondents are sent to the nominees' respective agency head for endorsement. A Membership Committee will make member selections for new voting members, which is reviewed and approved by the JOAG. The names and nomination materials are then sent to the Surgeon General for concurrence and appointment.

Senior Officer Advisor
A Senior Advisor to the JOAG, who must be an officer at the rank of 0-6 or above, is appointed by the Surgeon General. The Senior Advisor is an ex-officio member with a three-year term. The Senior Advisor is a consultant to the JOAG, who may advocate for, but not officially represent the JOAG.

Liaison, Commissioned Corps

The operating divisions and principal agencies of the Department of Health and Human Services each employ a commissioned officer or civilian who serves as the Commissioned Corps Liaison within their respective organization. The Liaisons are the principal program contact for operational Commissioned Corps matters, and they work closely with the Office of Commissioned Corps Operations. They also serve in the capacity of a personnel officer, providing information and assistance to commissioned officers assigned to their program.

Minority Officers Liaison Council

The Minority Officers Liaison Council (MOLC) provides advice and consultation on interests and concerns specific to minorities in the Commissioned Corps. Membership is for ethnic minority officers from PHS agencies and organizations staffed by PHS personnel.

Mission
The Minority Officers Liaison Council provides advice and consultation to the Surgeon General and, upon request, to agency and/or program heads of the Public Health Service, on issues relating to the professional practice and personnel activities relating to minorities in the PHS.

Objectives

The MOLC serves in a resource and advisory capacity to assist in the development, coordination and evaluation of activities related to ethnic minority officers it represents with the following objectives:
- Identifying and facilitating resolution of issues of concern as they relate to the ethnic minority officers.
- Assessing PHS personnel needs and assisting in meeting those needs through activities in recruitment, training, utilization and recognition of ethnic minority officers.
- Developing position papers, statistical reports and/or guidelines where appropriate, in order to advise and comment on matters relating to personnel issues of ethnic minority officers.
- Promoting the development and utilization of MOLC by the PHS and other governmental programs.
- Promoting all aspects of MOLC throughout the agencies and programs of the PHS.
- Providing liaison among ethnic minority officers within and among PHS components, and providing advice and consultation to the agency heads and operating programs upon request.

Membership

Composition. The Minority Officers Liaison Council is comprised of fulltime Commissioned Corps (CC) or Civil Service (CS) personnel. The Council includes two representatives from each of four ethnic minority committees/groups, as follows:
- American Indian/Alaskan Native Commissioned Officers Advisory Committee
- Asian Pacific American Officers Committee
- Black Commissioned Officers Advisory Group
- Hispanic Officers Advisory Committee

The MOLC may have from 4 to 8 voting members; at least two of those members must be assigned to a duty station 75 or more miles from the Washington, DC metropolitan area. Efforts must be made to ensure that the MOLC has broad representation from among all agencies, and does not consist entirely of one gender. At least one voting member must, at the time of appointment, have less than five years of professional experience. The MOLC shall not consist entirely of CC or entirely CS personnel. Members serve a term of two years, not to exceed a cumulative total of four years.

Nomination. Officers acting as Chair and Vice Chair of the four minority committees/groups serve as designated members to the MOLC. Of those designated members, officers to the MOLC will serve in the positions of Chair, Vice Chair, Secretary, and Recorder for a one-year term on a rotational schedule.

Music Ensemble

The USPHS Commissioned Corps Music Ensemble is the official PHS musician group at ceremonial and other occasions. It was formed in July 2000 under the sponsorship of the Scientist Professional Advisory Committee (SciPAC). The Scientist Chief Professional Officer (CPO) serves as the liaison between the Music Ensemble and the Office of the Surgeon General.

Mission
The Music Ensemble represents the Office of the Surgeon General and provides musical support for PHS, HHS and non-HHS sponsored events. It promotes esprit de corps within the Corps, and visibility of the Commissioned Corps within and outside of HHS.

Performance Venues
The Ensemble performs at ceremonies and events sponsored by the PHS, HHS and other Federal agencies. Awards ceremonies, promotion ceremonies, presentations by high ranking officials, official receptions, retirement ceremonies, special events, and memorial services are among the types of events at which the Ensemble performs. In addition, the Ensemble may perform at PHS-related venues. These include, among others, events sponsored by the Commissioned Officers Association of the USPHS, Anchor and Caduceus Society, and National Naval Medical Center. The Ensemble also seeks appropriate civilian venues at which to perform, both to provide community service and increase the visibility of the PHS.

Composition
The Ensemble is comprised of three groups:
- Choral Group
- Instrumental Wind Group
- Instrumental Chamber Group

The parent groups are located in the Washington, DC metropolitan area and are complemented by field units in various parts of the U.S. Each of the groups is capable of performing independently or in concert with one another.

Unlike most uniformed services where appointment to a musician Corps is the principal duty assignment, those officers who comprise the PHS Music Ensemble participate in this activity in addition to their regularly assigned duties. Membership in the Ensemble calls for a particular dedication to the PHS Commissioned Corps, yet it can be a highly rewarding experience for those who accept the challenge.

Basic Standards

Any active duty, ready Reserve, inactive Reserve or retired officer in good standing is eligible to become a member of the Music Ensemble. Prospective members should already have some music training and/or experience.

Officers are considered probationary members for the first six months of service in the Ensemble, after which they are eligible for full membership. Full membership is granted when the officer attains an acceptable level of musical proficiency; when the officer meets prescribed standards for attendance at rehearsals, practices and performances; and when the officer shows ongoing commitment to mission.

The officer members of the Ensemble volunteer their personal time and talent, to include a sometimes demanding schedule of rehearsals that are normally held during nonduty hours. Ensemble performances at official events are often held during duty hours, so supervisory support for the member is sought. Because they represent the Office of the Surgeon General, Ensemble members are expected to conduct themselves in a highly professional manner, maintain their uniforms in excellent condition, and to be thoroughly familiar with military protocol.

Oversight

The Office of the Surgeon General oversees the Ensemble in consultation with the Scientist CPO. An Executive Director, who is selected by the Office of the Surgeon General, administers the Ensemble and is responsible for all performance arrangements. The Executive Director and three Group Leaders form the Music Ensemble Executive Committee which provides ongoing supervision of Ensemble operations. Requests for an Ensemble performance are submitted to the Executive Director.

Professional Advisory Committee

Each of the eleven professional categories, as defined in the USPHS, has a Professional Advisory Committee (PAC). The Professional Advisory Committee provides advice on professional and personnel matters to its Chief Professional Officer (CPO) and the Surgeon General. Membership is representative of employees of PHS and other Federal agencies where officers are assigned. Membership on a PAC offers a PHS officer the opportunity to learn about issues and policies that affect them and their profession, as well as other officers. Because work is largely accomplished through subcommittees, officers can also become involved as a subcommittee member, which does not require formal membership on the PAC.

Mission
The Professional Advisory Committee (PAC) provides advice and consultation to the Surgeon General, through the Chief Professional Officer, on issues relating to the professional practice and personnel activities of those in the respective professional category, who are Civil Service employees or USPHS Commissioned Corps officers. The PAC provides similar advisory assistance to the Chief Professional Officer (CPO) and, upon request, to the agency and/or program heads of the Public Health Service and non-PHS agencies that routinely employ PHS personnel.

Objectives
The PAC serves in a resource and advisory capacity to assist in the development, coordination and evaluation of PHS professional activities with the following objectives:
- To identify and facilitate the resolution of issues related to the professional category.
- To assess professional personnel needs and assist in meeting those needs through activities in recruitment, training, utilization and recognition of professional category members.
- To develop position papers, statistical reports, and/or guidelines where appropriate, in order to advise and comment on matters relating to personnel and professional practice issues.
- To promote the development and utilization of subject professionals by the PHS and other government programs.
- To promote cooperation and communication among the subject professionals and health professionals in other disciplines.
- To promote all aspects of the subject professional category throughout the PHS agencies and other government programs.
- To provide liaison to professional disciplines within and among PHS components, and provide advice and consultation to the agency heads and operating programs upon request.

Relation to Organizations
In carrying out its responsibilities, the PAC operates in a staff capacity. It does not substitute for line management or in any way exercises the prerogatives of the respective agency programs.

Members are representative of all major PHS agencies/operating divisions (OpDivs) of HHS and non-HHS agencies where officers are assigned. While members are chosen from the respective agencies and organizations, they neither represent agency management nor speak for the agency. The members are knowledgeable professionals who represent a cross section of the interests, concerns, and responsibilities of the professionals in agencies staffed by PHS personnel.

PAC Designations
PAC names begin with the professional category, or modification thereto, as follows:
- Dental Professional Advisory Committee (DePAC)
- Dietitian Professional Advisory Committee (D-PAC)
- Engineer Professional Advisory Committee (EPAC)
- Environmental Health Officer Professional Advisory Committee (EHOPAC)
- Health Services Professional Advisory Committee (HS-PAC)
- Nursing Professional Advisory Committee (N-PAC)
- Pharmacist Professional Advisory Committee (PharmPAC)
- Physician Professional Advisory Committee (PPAC)
- Scientist Professional Advisory Committee (SciPAC)
- Therapist Professional Advisory Committee (TPAC)
- Veterinarian Professional Advisory Committee (VetPAC)

Membership
Composition and Term. The Professional Advisory Committee is comprised of both civilian and commissioned members within the particular professional category from a prescribed list of agencies. The PAC may have from 7 to 20 voting members; at least two of those members must be assigned to a duty station 75 or more miles from the Washington, DC metropolitan area. The PAC membership must include at least one Civil Service and one Commissioned Corps voting member, and at least one voting member must be an individual with fewer than five years experience as a professional. Efforts need to be made to ensure that the PAC does not consist entirely of one gender or race. The CPO is a non-voting ex officio member of the PAC. Members serve a term of three years, not to exceed a cumulative total of six years.

Nomination. Member terms are staggered so that approximately one-third of the members' terms expire annually. Each year, the PAC will solicit, through broadcast e-mail and newsletters, nominations (including self-nominations) for vacancies. The names of respondents are sent to the nominees' respective agency head for endorsement. The PAC and CPO will then identify, by name, highly qualified individuals whose names will be sent to the Surgeon General for approval.

Protocol Officer

A protocol officer is an officer or civilian who oversees the implementation of official protocol standards for an institution or organization. In the Federal government, the protocol officer provides fulltime management and support service to high ranking government officials, flag officers and to commands that are commanded by a flag rank officer (hereinafter referred to as the "superior officer"). The protocol officer advises the superior officer and staff on military customs and courtesies, tradition, organization and policy. Their responsibilities include detailed planning for visits by distinguished visitors (DVs), official travel, conferences, recognition programs, special ceremonies and official functions. The protocol officer also maintains a protocol library for the command.

A protocol officer serves as a representative of the superior officer or command to which assigned, and it is imperative that whatever actions are taken are consistent with established protocol and carried out as flawlessly as possible.

The uniformed services employ hundreds of protocol officers who receive specialized training in order to ensure that all activities are conducted professionally and in accordance with government, military and social protocol. In the military, the position of protocol officer is one of the more sensitive positions in a command—the ability of the command to manage events and projects that have high visibility will reflect favorably, or unfavorably, upon the leadership.

Background and Knowledge
Those who serve as a protocol officer should have certain basic qualifications. It is essential that the protocol officer have a comprehensive understanding of his/her own service and familiarity with other uniformed services—their history, mission, organization, and general operating procedures. A PHS protocol officer needs to have knowledge about the agencies to which PHS officers are assigned and, over time, have an acquaintance with the principal officials of those agencies.

The protocol officer is an authority on government, military and social customs, traditions, courtesies and protocol. To learn this well, protocol officers receive formal training provided by the uniformed service or a protocol school outside the service, and are expected to maintain proficiency through self-directed study.

Personal Qualities
The protocol officer must have a strong sense of integrity in his dealings with others and be capable of making good decisions at all times. If mistakes are made, the protocol officer must move ahead without making excuses. Through his actions, the protocol officer must attain a level of confidence by the superior officer.

There are certain attributes, which follow, that a protocol officer needs in order to carry out the position duties with proficiency.

Communication Skills. The protocol officer must be skilled in both verbal and written communication. Much depends on the maintenance of good interpersonal communications, and the ability of the protocol officer to listen well and communicate clearly with others is critical.

A protocol officer works directly with the superior officer, command leadership and principal staff, so a good communications relationship needs to be formed between the officer and the leadership—he must be comfortable in discussing any matter with the leadership on a one-on-one basis.

Cooperation and Teamwork. The protocol officer needs to be a leader in attitude and action. He must be able to work effectively with all persons, and be a conciliator who is sensitive to the motivations and needs of others. It is important to instill a sense of cooperation and teamwork among those involved in an event or project, so the officer needs to be a person who can bring others together in a common purpose.

Organization and Resourcefulness. The protocol officer should have an ability to properly organize and prioritize the myriad of details that accompany his duties. The ability to gather, review and disseminate information in an orderly way is critical to accomplishing the mission.

The effective protocol officer is also resourceful. He will have sufficient knowledge and experience to plan in advance for, and meet any contingency with competence. While most events or projects will require coordinated teamwork, a protocol officer must be ready to personally take whatever action is necessary to complete a project, even if such tasks might ordinarily be performed by others.

Appearance. The protocol officer must have an appearance that is in keeping with proper military appearance and bearing. The appearance of the protocol officer impacts significantly on the perception that others have of the superior officer and command. If a commissioned officer, one's uniforms are to be maintained in conformance with the highest uniform standards. Knowledge of the proper dress for different occasions is essential, both for himself and when he may be called upon to advise the leadership.

Readiness Force

The PHS Commissioned Corps Readiness Force (CCRF) was created in 1994 by the Office of the Surgeon General to improve the capability of the Department of Health and Human Services to respond to urgent public health emergencies. In 2003, the CCRF underwent a name change to the Office of Force Readiness and Deployment (OFRD). OFRD is one of four offices under the Office of the Surgeon General and it administers the readiness activities related to deployment of commissioned officers, as well as the civilian Medical Reserve Corps.

Mission
The stated mission of the OFRD is to provide public health leadership and expertise in times of extraordinary need during disasters, strife, or other public

health emergencies, in response to Federal, tribal, state, local or international requests. The PHS must be ready to respond to natural and intentional public health disasters. To that end, it is essential that PHS officers have the knowledge, training and preparation to quickly mobilize for any foreseeable type of disaster relief in the United States and abroad. Training should include provision for building interoperability—the ability to operate in concert with other uniformed service personnel. For these reasons, PHS officers must place a high premium on being personally and professionally prepared for any contingency.

Operations
Assistance Requests. Requests for Commissioned Corps assistance may be in response to any of the following:
- Public health challenges that exceed the capabilities of local, state or Federal resources.
- Public health requirements under the National Response Plan, of the Department of State and/or Agency for International Development, or during other declared emergencies.
- Critical technical public health requirements outside normal agency capabilities.
- Activation of the HHS Mass Immigration Plan.

Once the mission requirements are determined, OFRD will match the requirement against the qualifications of officers on that month's ready roster.

Activation Process. The process for activating Commissioned Corps deployments is a stepwise procedure, summarized as follows.
- Request for Assistance—OFRD evaluates the need and whether it will involve an appropriate utilization of commissioned officers.
- Request for Activation—OFRD submits a formal request for activation to the Surgeon General, who is briefed on the situation. If the Surgeon General concurs, and after notification of the Assistant Secretary for Health, ready rosters of officers are activated.
- Identification of Assets—Needs of the mission are matched with the capabilities of officers on the rotational ready roster, and individual officers are identified. When the requirements of the mission exceed the capability of a single ready roster, multiple rosters may be utilized.
- Deployment—Officers on the roster are contacted for confirmation of availability, which generally includes concurrence of the agency or OpDiv to which an officer is assigned. Travel orders and arrangements are prepared and officers are deployed to the situation.

There are seven rotational rosters, each of which has representation from all professional categories. Officers are on-call during the month that their roster is active. Officers must confirm their availability and the roster then represents the pool of officers that could be utilized to respond during that specific time period.

Basic Standards

All commissioned officers are required to meet the Basic level of force readiness. Standards for the Basic level are as follows.
- Health and Safety Standards—Disaster settings often require more than a person's usual physical exertion, involving lifting, carrying and walking, and working 12+ hour days. Healthcare workers are also at risk for exposure to infectious disease. Officers therefore need to be involved in an ongoing process of personal health maintenance and improvement. Officers are to obtain specified immunizations and Tuberculin Skin Test (PPD) screening, and record height and weight annually. The process also includes periodic monitoring of officers' health and well-being through a physical examination and medical history at least every five years.
- Physical Readiness Standards—These standards are to ensure that the physical capabilities of officers are consistent with their assignments. There are currently two physical fitness options for meeting the physical readiness standards annually: completion of the President's Challenge Physical Activity and Fitness Awards Program, or meeting or exceeding specified performance standards of a physical fitness test.
- Training and Professional Competency Standards—Officers must have a basic level of understanding in the areas of public health and deployment-response activities, have proficiency in basic life support measures, and maintain professional competency. This is accomplished through:
  - Completion of specified Web-based readiness training modules for the Basic level of force readiness.
  - Completion of, and maintain currency in, one of the following: American Heart Association Basic Life Support or Advanced Cardiac Life Support for Healthcare Providers, or the American Red Cross CPR/AED for the Professional Rescuer.
- Professional Competency—Healthcare providers must have and maintain a current unrestricted professional license, certification, or registration for his/her profession. Officers who wish to deploy in a clinical role (e.g., dentist, dietitian, nurse, pharmacist, physician, psychologist, social worker) must also practice a minimum of 112 hours per year in that role.
- Uniforms—Officers must have all required deployment uniforms.

Deployment Preparation

PHS deployments can cover a range of geographic and situational conditions. Officers should always keep at least one suitcase packed with items that would be useful in any type of deployment. Some general things should be kept in mind.
- Luggage should be sturdy and have a lock. Two pieces of luggage can be brought—one carry-on and one check-in bag. Do not pack more than you can carry, and keep at least one set of clothes, personal medications, and all professional equipment in the carry-on bag.

- Clothing and uniforms should be appropriate for the mission. Bring enough clothes and prescribed uniforms to last for 14 days, consistent with the weather and including a light rain jacket. Shoes should be comfortable, and also bring exercise clothes and shoes.
- Food and bottled water for one day's worth of emergency need should be carried in the carry-on bag. Possible food items may include items such as MREs (Meal, Ready-to-Eat), dehydrated food and cereal bars.
- Miscellaneous items to bring, in addition to personal care and toiletry items, include sun screen, sun glasses, insect repellent, sewing kit, shower shoes, small portable radio, reading materials, Zip Loc bags, and cash (automatic teller machines will not operate in settings with no power).

The chart in Appendix E provides a listing of suggested items to take on a deployment. Officers should modify it to meet individual needs that relate to the specific deployment.

Recruiter

There is an increasing need to recruit health care professionals for the U.S. Public Health Service, particularly in this time of national preparedness. In response, the PHS introduced the Associate Recruiter Program (ARP), whereby active duty, ready Reserve and retired officers can assist in recruiting highly qualified individuals for a career in the Commissioned Corps.

Associate Recruiter Program
The Office of Commissioned Corps Operations (OCCO) has a centralized, formal program for personnel recruitment. However, in order to supplement its recruitment program, OCCO sponsors the Associate Recruiter Program, which empowers commissioned officers to recruit health professionals for service in the PHS. The ARP is a volunteer program by which officers assist with recruitment, in addition to their regular duties. Although officers need not be in the ARP to perform recruitment activities, enrollment in the ARP allows recruiting efforts to be recognized by the PHS.

Duties. An Associate Recruiter informs colleagues and students about professional opportunities available in the Corps. They conduct recruitment presentations to interested and qualified individuals at work, colleges and universities, employment fairs, professional conferences and other appropriate venues. Presentations should be augmented with print and/or video materials.

Requirements. Officers must meet certain ARP requirements to remain in the program. These standards are as follows.
- Submit an ARP enrollment form.

- Accomplish at least two activities within a 12-month period. Activities must be recorded on an official form. Examples are the following:
  - Contact at least five potential PHS applicants or conduct a presentation to a group of five or more to talk about the Corps.
  - Spend a minimum of four hours in a recruiting booth at a national or regional meeting.
  - Precept a COSTEP, resident or extern for one month.
  - Visit a local high school for career day or class lecture to speak to students about opportunities in the USPHS.

Recognition. Officers wear the Associate Recruiter Badge on their uniform.

Surgeon General's Policy Advisory Council

The Surgeon General's Policy Advisory Council (SGPAC) constitutes a framework within which the Department of Health and Human Services (HHS) and other Federal agencies that utilize commissioned officers for providing advice to the Surgeon General (SG) and Deputy Surgeon General on policy matters related to the Commissioned Corps.

Objectives
The SGPAC is a resource and advisory group for the SG to evaluate policies affecting the Commissioned Corps, with the specific objectives of:
- Identifying policy issues that are of mutual concern to the SG and to the agencies.
- Advising the SG of potential impact on agencies of proposed Commissioned Corps policy and procedure issuances.
- Identifying and facilitating resolution of issues when conflicts of interest arise among different agencies.
- Serving as a forum for discussion of cross cutting issues that affect commissioned officers.

Membership and Authority
The SGPAC is comprised of a representative from all major HHS agencies/operating divisions and other agencies that are assigned PHS officers. SGPAC members are nominated by their agency and approved by the Surgeon General. Members must be at the senior grade (0-5) or equivalent Civil Service grade, and above.

In carrying out its responsibilities, the SGPAC operates in an advisory capacity. The SGPAC members speak on behalf of the agency they represent on policy issues related to the Commissioned Corps. However, members do not substitute for line management or in any way exercise the authorities of their respective operating programs, unless delegated by their programs.

SECTION V.

COMMUNICATIONS

Virtually every aspect of professional and service life involves both verbal and written communication. Effective interpersonal and organizational communications are vital to the proper functioning of a group and in promoting a positive "corporate image," whether a uniformed service, government institution or business entity.

> BUSINESS CARDS
> CALLS & CARDS
> CONVERSATION
> CORRESPONDENCE
> GREETINGS & INTRODUCTIONS
> PRESENTATIONS & SPEAKING
> TELECOMMUNICATIONS

Business Cards

All PHS officers should have a business/personal card. The card provides an efficient means for providing contact information and is a way for others to remember you. Because of its importance, the business card should reflect quality in every respect.

Specifications
The form of business cards can vary widely, but a commissioned officer's card is conservative by design. The card conforms to the standard size of 3½ by 2 inches, allowing it to fit into a business card holder. If not already set by the command authority, the overall appearance, texture and color of card stock and print characteristics need to be carefully selected. Print characteristics include the color of print, font (typeface, size and style), and whether the card

is printed, engraved, thermographed (raised print), embossed (the image is in relief, with or without ink), or some combination thereof.

Format
The format of the military business card may vary. Unless a format is specified, the officer's institutional logo (e.g., Department of Health and Human Services or agency to which assigned) is typically located in the upper left corner of the card. PHS officers may also elect to use the USPHS logo alone or in concert with the institution logo; if both are used, place the logos in upper opposing corners of the card. No more than two logos should be used.

An officer's name and academic degree may be centered. Rank and uniformed service designation, or position, can be placed on the next line or in the lower right corner, as appropriate. Some positions may require, or the officer may prefer, that rank appear on the first line preceding one's name. When using that format, there should be no trailing professional credentials. In addition to duty station address and telephone number, business cards will typically include facsimile number and e-mail address in the lower corner(s).

Note that honorifics (e.g., Dr., Mr., Ms., etc.) are not used on business cards, in contrast to social cards. A nickname may be included only if well established (e.g., Admiral John ("Jack") Kearns).

Sample Business Card

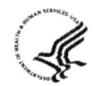

James E. Ford, Ph.D.
Captain, U.S. Public Health Service
Director, Division of Drug Information

(301) 555-1000
FORDJ@FDA.GOV

FOOD AND DRUG ADMINISTRATION
5600 FISHERS LANE, ROOM 8B32
ROCKVILLE, MD 20852

Purpose
The business card is properly used as follows:
- to give professional or uniformed service identification information to another individual, such as a colleague, business client or contact, or patient;
- as a cover attachment to official documents being sent to others, to identify the sender;
- as an enclosure with a business gift, to identify the sender if not well known to the recipient (although a calling card or gift card may be preferable);
- occasionally (though not recommended) to serve as a medium for brief messages on the back.

Providing Card
Following are a few guidelines for the use of business cards.
- Provide only crisp, clean, and up-to-date cards.
- Provide your card to those who have shown an interest in receiving or exchanging such information.
- Do not offer your card to those who are superior in rank, unless there is evident interest in receiving your card.
- Do not offer your card to unknown persons you happen to meet, unless there is evident interest in receiving your card.
- When at a business meeting with others whom you do not know, cards may be exchanged at the beginning of the meeting.
- Do not leave a pile of cards or scatter them about at a large general meeting or other such gathering.
- Generally, withhold giving cards at a strictly social event. However, if offered privately and not at a dinner table, it is alright.
- For close friends and those who are ill, a gift card or personal note is preferred as an enclosure with flowers or a gift.
- When used as an attachment or enclosure, it is preferred that you write a note on the front or back (write "over" on the front) of the card. If the recipient is someone you know well, line out the printed name and sign your given (first) name.

Receiving Card
When someone gives you their business card, reciprocate with a card of your own. When handed their card, take time to review it and thank the person for giving you this information. This is particularly important in the international arena, where the business/name card and the protocol that surrounds it has considerable importance. It is always improper to receive a business card and simply place it in your pocket.

Business cards have an importance that far outweighs their minimal cost and one should not scrimp on procuring high quality cards.

Calls & Cards

Although PHS officers do not typically make official and social calls, it is important to have some familiarity with these military customs.

Official Calls
Upon arrival at a new duty station, a military officer officially reports for duty to the commanding officer (CO), carrying the orders that effected the transfer of duty. In addition, unless dispensed with by the senior authority, a courtesy call is made by the officer on the commanding officer (CO) in his/her office.

These calls last about 10 to 15 minutes and afford the CO and officer an opportunity to meet and learn about each other in a less formal meeting. Alternatively, at large stations where many officers are posted and time constraints preclude a personal meeting, an arriving officer may instead be introduced to the CO at the first officer staff meeting. The new officer may follow-up with a brief courtesy call, by appointment.

Social Calls
Within two weeks of reporting for duty, social calls are made by an arriving officer and his/her spouse at the home of the commanding officer, who in turn returns the call to the officer's home. The new officer should limit the visit to 15 to 30 minutes unless requested to stay longer and, if expected (check with the executive or protocol officer), leave a calling/personal card upon departure. Though no longer common, these formal at-home visits are still the custom at some military stations and in Europe.

The custom that is in wide use today is for the commanding or other senior officer and his spouse to periodically host one or more receptions, occasionally at their residence, where hospitality is extended to officers of the command and their spouses. These functions are usually considered "calls made and paid," meaning that those in attendance need not reciprocate with an invitation to the CO and his spouse. At large gatherings, arriving officers and their spouses may be announced to the commanding officer and his spouse, who greet each guest. When departing the reception, those attending should thank the host and hostess if they are not occupied with other guests. A short thank you note may also be sent.

Calling Cards
Calling cards are used for social calls and for making official calls in a foreign country. The military calling/personal card conforms to the standard size of 3½ by 2 inches. The officer's rank (spelled out), first name, middle initial and surname are placed in the center of the card, followed by the service designation in the lower right corner (no logo). The personal card may also be used as an enclosure with gifts.

When assigned to a foreign country, an officer is advised to contact the protocol officer of the American Embassy for guidance on the policy regarding official calls. Calling or attaché cards should be prepared in advance of the change in duty station. There is a prescribed format for attaché cards, and officers may elect either to print both sides of the card, one side in English and the other in the language of the country to which assigned, or print two sets of cards, with English on one set and the other language on the second set.

Military calling cards are conservative in design. The color of card stock is white or ecru (light cream), with black lettering.

Conversation

"There can be no doubt that of all the accomplishments prized in modern society, that of being agreeable in conversation is the very first. ...It is agreed among us that people must meet frequently, both men and women, and that not only is it agreeable to talk, but that it is a matter of common courtesy to say something, even when there is hardly anything to say."

From the Introduction to
The Principles of the Art of Conversation,
by J.P. Mahaffy, 1891.

Effective communication in business, the professions and uniformed services is essential to success. Most communication is verbal, involving the art of speaking and listening, using words as the primary medium.

There are two principal types of verbal communication—official and social. In work situations, conversation may be more technical and to the point, yet under normal circumstances is pleasant with due deference to rank or seniority. Rank has its privileges and when very senior personnel are present, the general rule is to allow senior officers to lead. This should not stifle candid discussions of a business nature by more junior staff.

Social settings provide an opportunity to engage in "small talk" which is also pleasant but which has less import. Social conversation breaks down certain barriers and provides latitude to the range of topics that can be discussed, as long as such discussions are cordial and not injurious to others or yourself.

Military officers adhere to a certain protocol with regard to their verbal discourse with other officers.

- For conveying greetings from senior officers, use the form "Admiral Williams presents his compliments to Commander Garcia and says…" (a junior officer does not "present his compliments" to a senior). For making an official or social call upon a senior officer, a junior officer correctly says "Admiral Williams, I came to pay my respects" or "Inform the Admiral that Commander Garcia would like to pay his respects."
- Senior officers who "direct," "desire," or "suggest" that something be done to junior officers are, in effect, giving a directive or order. Junior officers may only "recommend" an action or "request" senior officers to act.
- Senior officers "call" or "direct attention" to something, whereas junior officers "invite attention."
- Senior officers acknowledge information provided by junior officers by responding "very well," whereas junior officers acknowledge a direct order with "yes, Sir."

Effective Speaking and Listening

Words can have many meanings, but if they are properly communicated and received, mutual understanding will occur. Other factors enter into verbal communication, however, and include the pitch, tone, volume and inflection of your voice; nonverbal forms of communication such as body language; and, the perception which the listener places on the message. In other words, how you say (and when listening, how you interpret) the spoken word can be as important as what is actually stated. Persons who are cognizant of these factors tend to be more adept in their official and social dealings. Those who also have a good conversational style have an added advantage—they can move through subjects with greater ease, making themselves more interesting and therefore more closely listened to by others.

The effectiveness in conveying your thoughts can depend, to a large extent, on the speaking tools you employ and conversational etiquette you show towards others. For instance:

- Articulate words with an agreeable pitch, tonal quality, tempo or rate of speech, and volume of sound. Give expression to the words through appropriate variations in those vocal characteristics, so that real interest in the subject is evident to the listener. Avoid contrived speech characteristics. This does not preclude the need to modify one's normal speech pattern in appropriate circumstances; for example, a military leader who is trying to rally support for a mission will modify his delivery in a way that commands attention and gains acceptance of the message.

- Use proper grammar and a good working vocabulary that is conversational, natural and suited to your style. Avoid the following: filler words such as "uh" or "you know;" slang or words that are of passing fashion such as "you guys" (particularly when addressing men *and* women); technical jargon; profanity; prejudicial ethnic or religious terms; and words that are considered sexist.

- Think before you speak. Do not place another person in an uncomfortable position by what you say. Be mindful of the timing and appropriateness of subject matter, in terms of both the context of the conversation and who you are speaking with.

- Be alert to signs of boredom in listeners and adjust accordingly. Do not dominate a conversation.

- Do not interrupt others who are speaking, particularly those who are senior in rank, with corrections of their grammar, injection of words or phrases the speaker is searching for (unless it is apparent that the person needs assistance), or with the finish to a speaker's story.

- Show interest in speaking and listening through good body language. Always greet others with a firm handshake. Stand or sit with posture comfortably erect. Give complete attention to those with whom you are

conversing—maintain good eye contact, avoid the "glazed" eye look or allowing your eyes to wander.
- Maintain good listening habits through concentration on the *thought* being conveyed. Take account of the speaker's choice of words and gestures used in conveying the thought. Occasionally, a deficient speaker or uninteresting subject will place impediments to effective listening. However, the effective listener overcomes these barriers by recognizing his responsibility to be attentive to the speaker and what could be potentially important information. A method of enhancing one's interest and displaying it to the speaker is to make listening responses such as asking questions and nodding affirmatively. A note of caution regarding the latter behavior, however—leaders are not appreciative of junior officers who try to garner favor simply by appearing always to be in agreement with the senior officer.

Correspondence

The impression of you as an individual and the uniformed service you represent will be made by both the form and content of your written communications. While e-mail is often employed in place of structured styles of written communication, it is important to forego the ease of an e-mail when a more formal approach is called for. In whatever form, written correspondence that is properly formatted, grammatically correct and which effectively conveys your thoughts is an important component in the success of your work life. Not only is the ability to write well a valuable asset, it is often essential given the specialized work that is often performed.

Purpose
Types of official correspondence include e-mail, internal memoranda, business letters, letters of reference, letters of introduction, notes and reports. While the substance of these documents varies, all serve the purpose of communicating thought. That thought may be to inform, initiate action or record an event. Unlike direct verbal communication, the sender of a written document does not have real-time feedback from the recipient and, thus, the writer must be certain that the intended thought is clearly elucidated.

The type of document to be used depends on how formal or official the content is and whether the document is being sent internally or outside of the organization. The military letter conveys a sense of formality that may be warranted when writing to a very high ranking senior officer. A memorandum is less formal and may include acronyms that are commonly used within the organization; however, the format of the memorandum is often more standardized than a letter.

Appearance & Stationery

The overall appearance of official documents has an immediate impact on the reader's perception of the sender and may also influence how the message is received. Factors which combine to form a paper document's appearance include the stationery used, neatness, and format of those elements that comprise the document. The use of text embellishments such as character bolding or headings enhances the appearance as well as readability of documents.

Official stationery is ordinarily prescribed in terms of letterhead and print characteristics. Paper is of good quality bond, with a basis weight of 20 to 22 lb. Standard Business and up to 24 lb. Executive, with a rag or fiber content of at least 25%. Paper comes in various sizes, but most frequently in standard sizes of 8½" by 11" Standard; and, 7¼" by 10½" Executive for hand- or typewritten correspondence that is more personal in nature. Corresponding envelopes are commonly Commercial No. 10, 4⅛" by 9½", requiring two parallel folds of the business letter; and Executive, 3⅞" by 7½", requiring two parallel folds. Envelopes also come in the standard size of 3⅝" by 6½" for very brief notes.

Composition

Well written communications include those that are logically constructed, keeping in mind the purpose and intent. For lengthy documents, an outline is useful in organizing your thoughts—concepts may be arranged from the most to least important, chronologically, or in some other systematic approach. The outline should begin with the purpose of the communication and lead to a clear conclusion, recommendation or call for action. Make a determination regarding the need for a review of background material or research on a subject, and accomplish this task before proceeding further; the outline is then revised accordingly. State the more salient points early and provide any supporting material. Sentences should be clear and concise, grammatically correct and have no spelling errors. Word selection and usage are important—a conversational style is usually considered best, avoiding multisyllabic or overly technical terms and stilted phraseology. A written draft should be reviewed and revised as often as necessary until it is satisfactory.

A critical aspect of any document is the tone it conveys. Military correspondence that has a professional, yet friendly tone is generally better received and more effective in achieving its intended objective. All documents should convey a sense of credibility and an interest in the reader's perspective. Interoffice memoranda and e-mail provide an efficient method of transmitting ideas to your colleagues, and may be less formal and more to the point that a business letter.

Letter and Memoranda Elements

Official correspondence has specified elements which, for letters and memoranda, are compared and summarized as follows:

LETTER	MEMORANDUM*
Date	Date: line
Inside address	To: line
No From: line	From: line
Subject introduced in first paragraph	Subject: line
Salutation	*No* salutation
Indent paragraphs of text	Left justify all text
Complimentary close	*No* complimentary close
Signature	Signature
Signature block	*No* signature block

*Align left margin with centerline of the letterhead seal.

Letter Elements *(see Composite Letter, page 99)*

There are standard elements to official correspondence.

Date. For a *letter,* the date is centered two or more lines below the letterhead, taking into account the overall length of the letter. Both civilian and military practice is to use the sequence of month-day-year with a comma after the day (e.g., October 15, 2007).

For a *memorandum,* uniformed services use day-month-year without punctuation (e.g., 15 October 2007). If the month is abbreviated without punctuation, the year is indicated by the last two digits (e.g., 15 Oct 07).

Declarations/Notations *(optional).* Special mailing declarations and on-arrival notations are next, placed flush with the left margin, entirely capitalized (e.g., REGISTERED MAIL, or CONFIDENTIAL).

Inside Address. The inside address should begin with the person's full name, preceded by an honorific (e.g., CDR, Dr., Mr., Ms.) or followed by an academic or professional degree (in which case the honorific is not used). The person's position or functional title, duty station or business name, and address follow on successive lines. If the letter is addressed to an institution and an attention line is needed, place it on the line following the duty station/company name. The envelope is normally addressed the same as the inside address.

Subject. In an official letter, the subject is introduced in the first paragraph. If needed for referencing purposes, however, place a subject line before the salutation. Words such as Subject:, Reference:, RE:, or Re: may be used.

Salutation. The salutation "Dear" plus an honorific—a person's personal or professional title (may abbreviate), or uniformed service title (spelled out)—and addressee's surname is standard.

When on a first name basis, the writer may use "Dear" and the person's given name. Note, however, that for form letters and when a higher ranking commissioned officer writes to a lower rank officer who is well known to the senior officer, the sender may instead line-out the recipient's typewritten surname and handwrite that officer's given name above the surname.

Text. The body of a letter is single-spaced, with one space between paragraphs. For brief letters, one and one-half or double spacing can be used. A minimum of two or three lines of text warrant a continuation sheet. There are numerous formats used for continuation sheets, among which are:
- Enter the page number at the top of each page with spaced hyphens
  - 2 -
- Place the word "Page" and the page number flush with the left margin
  Page 2
- Place "Page" and page number flush left, followed with a spaced hyphen and the addressee's honorific and name
  Page 2 - LT Thomas Kelly

Complimentary Close. The complimentary close is placed about two lines below the text.

Military officials tend to use a more formal term. A customary way to close written correspondence is for senior officers to use "Respectfully," when writing to junior personnel. Junior officers corresponding with senior officers close with "Very respectfully." When less formality is acceptable, officers can abbreviate and use "R", "V/R" or "V/r". There are other polite closes for a business letter:

    Formal: *Very respectfully yours, Respectfully yours, Very truly yours,*
    Less Formal: *Very sincerely yours, Sincerely yours, Most Sincerely,*
                  Sincerely,
    Informal and Personal: *Cordially yours, Yours cordially, Kindest regards,*
                         Best regards, Regards, Best wishes,

Signature Block. The signature block is aligned vertically with, and placed three to five lines below the complimentary close. The writer's name, followed by professional degrees, is placed on the first line of the signature block (degrees are *not* included with the person's written signature). In business, the writer's functional title follows on the second line. For commissioned officers, the writer's rank and service designation follow on the second line, with his/her position placed on the third line.

Note that in the uniformed services, the officer's name is printed in *all* capital letters for official (e.g., departmental directives) letters and memoranda.

Closing Data. Closing data such as the name or initials of those persons who draft a letter, if different from the signer, typically are placed only on the office file copy of a letter. Attachment or enclosure information is placed flush with the left margin, after the signature block. The document attached/enclosed should be specified and, if more than one, should be numbered.

Letter Formats *(see Composite Letter, below)*
There are several accepted formats for preparing an official letter. The following are brief descriptions of the forms commonly in use.
Full Block Form. The full block form of a letter simply means that all letter elements, discussed above, are begun flush with the left margin.
Modified Block Form. The modified block form of a letter follows the full block form, *except* that the date, complimentary close and signature begin at the center or to the right-of-center of the page.
Modified Semi-Block Form. This form follows the modified block form, except that the first word of each paragraph of the text is indented.
Executive Form. This uses the modified semi-block format, *except* that the inside address, flush left, is placed below the signature block.

Composite Letter, Modified Block Form
This or the Semi-Modified Block Form are preferred in the uniformed services and Federal government.

DEPARTMENT OF HEALTH & HUMAN SERVICES
PUBLIC HEALTH SERVICE
OFFICE OF THE SURGEON GENERAL
WASHINGTON, DC 20201

July 15, 2008   (Date)

Josephine Smith, M.D.
Director   (Inside Address)
National Cancer Institute
9000 Rockville Pike
Bethesda, MD 20894

Dear Dr. Smith: (Salutation)

This is to confirm my presentation on Promoting the Nation's Health, to be given at the National Cancer Institute on July 27, 2008.

                    Sincerely,   (Complimentary Close)

(Signature Block)   Richard H. Carmona, M.D., M.P.H.
                     VADM, USPHS
                     United States Surgeon General

Greetings & Introductions

This section covers civilian and military greetings and introductions. For uniformed service practice, refer also to the Section, Military Courtesy & Protocol, Address & Greeting. Upon first meeting someone, the impression you convey impacts significantly on your future relationship. It is therefore important in dealing with uniformed service personnel, business associates and the public that you greet and address them, and make introductions cordially and properly.

Addressing Others

As a general rule, persons whom you first meet should be addressed by an honorific such as Mr., Ms., Mrs., or with a person's rank or professional title such as Commander, Doctor, Reverend, Senator, and the person's surname (last name). You should continue to address a person in this manner until he/she says that you may use their given (first) name or you become familiar enough with each other that use of the first name is acceptable.

Within most organizations today, first names are used among employees, with a title and person's last name reserved for more senior persons by age or executive rank. If you are on a first name basis and see a senior colleague accompanied by an outside person, however, you should address that colleague by rank or title and his last name.

The terms "sir" and "ma'am" are proper forms of address within uniformed services. "Madam" and "Madame" are appropriate as a title in officialdom (e.g., "Madam Chairperson") and in addressing untitled women who are citizens in certain other countries. Refer to the table "Forms of Address" on page 102 for a listing of proper forms of verbal and written address for civilian government officials.

Greetings

You always rise, step toward a visitor and remain standing when greeting or being introduced to that person. Similarly, when other than your co-workers, stand and welcome visitors and senior officials to your office.

Greet the other person cordially, with a pleasant demeanor. If you already know the person, something such as "How are you?" is said, and you may want to shake hands. Unless you are close personal friends, your response to such a greeting should be limited to something like "Fine, thanks, and you?" even if you are not doing very well. When being introduced to someone new, offer your hand in a comfortably firm handshake—a man need not wait for a woman to first offer her hand, as was previously the custom. If the palm of your hand is moist, subtly wipe it dry before a handshake. Ordinarily, a glove is removed prior to shaking hands.

After introductions are made, persons should say a few words of greeting to one another, such as "How do you do?" or "It's nice to meet you." A few pleasantries help to relax everyone, and any business should be initiated only after all participants have been seated and given a few minutes to become accustomed to the surroundings.

Introductions

Making introductions is a life-long endeavor that should come naturally. Whether at a meeting or social function, it is normally the host's responsibility to greet and introduce people. If a person's name is not clearly heard, you should ask that the name be repeated; and, if the host errs in introducing you, it is usually a good idea to affably correct the mistake. Always introduce an acquaintance whom only you know, if that person is with you or joins you during a group conversation. When introducing a spouse, use his/her first name (e.g., "Lieutenant Walsh, I would like you to meet my husband, Doug").

If you forget a person's name while making introductions and that person does not introduce himself, apologetically (but without embarrassment) admit your lapse of recall. If you perceive that a person making introductions has forgotten your name or you are not introduced, you should introduce yourself to the others present.

The proper manner of making introductions can be remembered if a few guidelines are kept in mind. You should introduce:
- a lower ranking person *to* a higher ranking person;
- a business colleague *to* an outside associate;
- a younger person *to* an older person;
- a family member *to* a business associate or colleague;
- all else being equal, a man *to* a woman.

The simplest way is to first name the person given preference. For example, "Admiral Carmona, I would like you to meet Captain Brad Johnson, our Director of Human Resources." Alternatively, reverse the sequence and emphasize the preposition "to." For example, "Captain Johnson, may I introduce you *to* Admiral Carmona, the Surgeon General."

As shown in these examples, it is important to provide descriptive information about a person when making introductions.

Introductions in a receiving line are the responsibility of the host, the guest who is queued in the waiting line, and/or a staff person assigned to facilitate introductions. At larger functions, when as a guest you may not be readily known by the host, you introduce yourself giving your name and identifier information (e.g., organizational position and affiliation). If a staff person is assisting, he will greet you, take your name and introduce you to the host who, in turn, introduces you to the next person receiving you or a guest of honor, if present. As the host, you should greet guests with a smile, a warm handshake and a pleasant remark.

Proper forms of address to use for government officials are given in the following table.

FORMS OF ADDRESS
CIVILIAN GOVERNMENT OFFICIALS*

Person	Written Address Introductions	Salutation	Conversation
FEDERAL			
President	The President The White House	Dear Mr. President	Mr. President or Sir
Vice-President	The Vice-President Old Executive Office Bldg.	Dear Mr. Vice-President	Mr. Vice-President or Mr. Clark or Sir
Cabinet Member	The Honorable David Clark Secretary of HHS	Dear Mr. Secretary or Dear Sir	Mr. Secretary or Secretary Clark or Mr. Clark
Senator	The Honorable David Clark U.S. Senate	Dear Senator Clark or Dear Sir	Senator or Senator Clark
Representative	The Honorable David Clark U.S. House of Represent.	Dear Mr. Clark or Dear Sir	Mr. Clark or Representative Clark
House Speaker	The Honorable David Clark Speaker of the H. of Repr.	Dear Mr. Speaker or Dear Sir	Mr. Speaker or Mr. Clark
Chief Justice	The Chief Justice The Supreme Court	Dear Mr. Chief Justice or Dear Sir	Mr. Chief Justice or Sir
Associate Justice	Mr. Justice Clark The Supreme Court	Dear Mr. Justice or Dear Justice Clark or Dear Sir	Mr. Justice or Justice Clark or Sir
Ambassador	The Honorable David Clark American Ambassador	Dear Mr. Ambassador or Dear Amb. Clark or Dear Sir	Mr. Ambassador or Ambassador Clark or Mr. Clark or Sir
STATE/LOCAL			
Governor	The Honorable David Clark Governor of Rhode Island	Dear Governor or Dear Governor Clark or Dear Sir	Governor or Governor Clark or Sir
Senator	The Honorable David Clark Rhode Island Senate	Dear Senator Clark or Dear Sir	Senator or Senator Clark; or Sir
Mayor	The Honorable David Clark Mayor of Newport	Dear Mr. Mayor or Mayor Clark; or Dear Sir	Mr. Mayor or Mayor Clark or Your Honor
Judge	The Honorable David Clark Judge, Superior Court	Dear Judge Clark	Mr. Justice or Judge Clark

*Substitute "Madam" in place of "Mr." or "Sir" for a woman official.

Presentations & Speaking

Most commissioned officers are called upon to make prepared presentations as a part of their position. As the speaker, you need to optimize your preparation, delivery and stage presence in order to effectively present a message. This not only helps in promoting your ideas, but fulfills the responsibility you have to provide credible information to those in attendance. Because public speaking conveys an "image" about the speaker and the uniformed service you represent, speaking ability can play a prominent role in one's advancement within the service. It is therefore worth the effort to work on improving your speaking skills.

Preparation
It is very important to thoroughly prepare before any presentation.
- Your presentation should be well organized by having a clear introduction and purpose or thesis, a body that focuses on the salient points you want to make, and an ending that provides a summary of the main points and conclusions.
- The text should be logically and concisely constructed. Utilize concrete examples and statistical data to illustrate and support your statements. Avoid rambling thoughts and statements.
- The language you use should be kept relatively simple, and terminology should be readily understandable to the audience.
- Practice your presentation in front of a mirror and, if possible, record your presentation. Listen carefully for voice characteristics; you will want to articulate words with good diction and an agreeable pitch, tonal quality, tempo or rate of speech, and volume of sound. Observe body movements—notice your posture, facial expressiveness, and arm and hand gestures. Work on problem areas and re-record yourself to determine if improvements are evident. If possible, conduct a "dry run" in the presence of a colleague.
- If you are using slides or other visual aids, incorporate them into your practice session. Make sure the visuals are properly sequenced and correspond with what you are saying, that they truly add substance to the presentation, are professional in appearance, and are large enough to be read at the back of the meeting room.
- Ensure that you finish the presentation within set time constraints.
- If not already known, familiarize yourself with the background and expectations of the audience so that, with this knowledge, you are more comfortable when speaking before them.
- Visit the meeting room beforehand to familiarize yourself with the setting, and to check on the working order and use of audiovisual equipment.

- Finally, use mental imagery to visualize yourself making the presentation, effectively and with confidence. Visualize this as a positive experience.

Delivery

The style of delivery may vary with the type of meeting. However, certain general statements can be made.
- Take a slow, deep breath and mentally calm yourself. Begin by thanking the person who introduced you and, if appropriate, greeting distinguished guests, including senior officers of note, and then the audience.
- Establish rapport with the audience. For instance, open with remarks or a humorous anecdote that relates yourself or the subject of the presentation with the audience or the meeting location.
- Use proper grammar and a good working vocabulary that is natural and suited to your style. Avoid the following: hesitations; filler words/phrases such as "uh" or "you know;" slang or words that are of passing fashion; and lingo or technical jargon unless appropriate for the audience.
- Unless giving a formal speech, it is usually best to use cards or papers on which key thoughts and phrases are written in outline form, rather than utilize a complete manuscript. Highlighting the outline or using margin notes can be helpful in identifying places in the presentation where more verbal emphasis is indicated.
- Visually, you should slowly pan over the audience, breaking regularly to make eye contact with individual members of the audience.
- Your voice should be confident and well modulated. Avoid being monotonal. Appropriate variations in pitch, tempo and volume of your voice make your thoughts more convincing and interesting to listen to.
- When using visual aids, use a pointer to indicate specific items on the visual that correspond with the content of your presentation, and speak to the audience (not toward the visual) whenever possible.
- If you take audience questions in a large room without the benefit of floor microphones, you should first repeat the question so that everyone may hear it.
- End the presentation on a "solid" or uplifting note.

Stage Presence

There are certain tips that may be helpful to keep in mind.
- Aside from greater visibility, standing and/or using a podium will impart more authority, control and formality to the meeting.
- Good body language is particularly important. Confidence and poise are conveyed by projecting a calm and friendly facial disposition, and maintaining an erect, but relaxed posture. Gesturing of the arms and hands is very effective if it is natural, sincere and not overdone. Avoid nervous mannerisms such as fidgeting with your hands.

- Always have a handkerchief available to use when you are about to cough or sneeze; simply cover your mouth with it and turn your head away from the audience and microphone. Avoid having pocket coins or jewelry that might jingle when you move.
- An authoritative personal appearance is important. You should always be well groomed and dressed in proper uniform that is clean and pressed.

Introducing the Speaker
The introduction of a speaker should be brief and upbeat. As the introducer, you should acquaint the audience with the speaker, mentioning significant aspects of his/her background and accomplishments (personalize this information when possible). Relate the reason for, or content of the presentation to the audience and pique their interest in what the speaker is about to say.

Immediately following the address, you should thank the speaker and comment on the excellence (or informative nature, etc.) of the presentation. If this also concludes the meeting program, thank the audience for their attendance at the function.

Telecommunications

E-mail, cell phone and telephone manners have a decided impact on the perception others have about one's professionalism and duty station. Communications that are handled intelligently, in a helpful and professional manner, show that you care about the other party and have leadership character.

Electronic Mail
E-mail is probably the leading method for daily communications due to its convenience and efficiency. E-mail has largely replaced telephonic communication, because those you try to reach by telephone may be unavailable to answer the phone. While a telephone conversation has the advantage of being interactive, it is also clear that some individuals prefer a less personal approach to communicate, and e-mail fulfills that preference. Although there are electronic document systems for sending written forms through a chain of command for approval, an e-mail generally lacks that capability when documents require a "Through:" line. When using e-mail, keep in mind the following.
- Use Discretion – E-mail is legally considered government property when utilized on the job. When composing an e-mail, be mindful of what you write—an e-mail is a permanent record that can easily be forwarded to others and therefore lacks assurance of confidentiality.

- Be Clear – Be sure that an e-mail conveys the message you intend, because it is not accompanied by body language or real time feedback from the recipient. Always review an e-mail before sending it. In some cases, it is advised that you delay sending an e-mail that may need further consideration and/or editing.
- Use Military Protocol – When sending an e-mail to senior personnel, use proper salutations and closings when appropriate.
- Use Appropriately – Unless necessary for archival purposes, e-mail is not recommended for very lengthy, complex or confidential information, and should not be for mail that is angry, critical or terse. Know when to opt for sending or attaching a properly formatted document which is usually perceived as more respectful or holding more importance, or opting to talk with a person directly or by telephone.
- Check Content – An e-mail reflects upon the sender, so make a good impression by proof reading the e-mail and using the computer software's spelling and grammar checks and its thesaurus feature.

Cellular Phone

Cell phones are a great technological advance that has become endemic in our daily lives. When used without regard for others, though, a cell phone becomes an annoyance and reflects poorly on the user. The following are some tips to keep in mind.
- Be Considerate – The cell phone ring tones from incoming calls are an unwelcome disturbance in certain settings. Turn off the phone or use the silent or vibrate mode in enclosed public places such as auditoriums, libraries, restaurants, theaters, and places of worship.
- Use Appropriately – In addition to enclosed public places, do not place or receive cell phone calls during business meetings. Avoid taking nonofficial calls in the presence of others when on duty time, since to do so may convey rudeness. If you must take a call in such settings, however, excuse yourself and keep your phone conversation brief.
- Use Discretion – Unless related to the business at hand, always converse in a low voice and, if a private matter, away from others who are in close proximity. When placing a call to someone else's cell phone during duty hours, it is a good practice to first ask if it is okay to talk with the person.

Telephone
- Answering – Answer the phone by the third ring with your rank and surname and, if appropriate, title (not simply "Hello"). Place a caller on hold at most about 40 seconds, and then check back periodically if prolonged. When transferring a call, give the caller the referral name and telephone number.
- Placing Calls – Whenever possible place your own calls, especially to senior officers. If you expect a lengthy discussion, provide the other

person with the purpose of your call and ask if they have sufficient time at the moment or if another time is more convenient. If disconnected, it is always the caller's responsibility to call back regardless of the cause.
- Other Guidelines – Return calls promptly, within the same day. If going to someone's office and that person is on the telephone, do not enter unless you are motioned in; and, if in someone's office who must take a call and you are motioned to stay, read or look elsewhere during the call. When ending an official call, thank the other person by name; for military personnel, state their rank and, optionally, surname ("Thank you, Commander Johnston").
- Conference Calls – Prepare ahead by locating a room with minimal or no background noise to receive the call. Be present early so that conferees can be connected ahead of time, if necessary, and introduce yourself when you begin speaking. If there is background noise or you need to speak to colleagues in the room off-record, use the mute button on the telephone.

SECTION VI.

MEETINGS

Meetings are endemic in government and the uniformed services, as well as in business. Meetings take many forms and are called for various purposes. They serve the needs of the organization and are a forum for participants. The effectiveness of a meeting relates directly to the skills of the chairperson and those in attendance. This Section provides guidance on optimizing one's personal effectiveness in meetings.

> THE CHAIRPERSON
> THE PARTICIPANTS
> OFFICE APPOINTMENTS
> CONVENTIONS
> PARLIAMENTARY PROCEDURE

Effective meetings are essential to proper management of any corporate entity. Meetings are called for the purposes of planning activities, briefings, providing information, solving problems and making decisions, or combination thereof. Types of meetings include the impromptu meeting in a colleague's office, appointments or scheduled meetings with others, regular policy or staff meetings, interdepartmental meetings, briefings, senior officer meetings and so on.

While the person who conducts a meeting is usually the most visible, each person at the meeting is on view. As a participant and officer, you are compared to, and evaluated by those in attendance on the basis of your mannerisms, how you think, and generally how you handle yourself and interact with others—in other words, you are judged on the basis of personal qualities and professional competence. Meetings are therefore important in not only furthering the work of the organization, but can be an important determinant in whether you advance and achieve your potential within the Commissioned Corps.

The Chairperson

The individual who leads a meeting sets the direction and tone of the proceedings, and has the responsibility to exercise control in a way that fosters and maintains productive communication among the participants. The degree of control will depend on the meeting purpose, agenda and attendees. For the uninitiated, this can be a challenge when controversial issues are before the group, while giving due deference to senior officers. It is therefore important that the chairperson be capable and knowledgeable, and someone in whom the participants have confidence. There are certain things to keep in mind when chairing a meeting.

Pre-Meeting
- The reason for calling the meeting and the objectives to be met should be clear. Select the persons to be invited as meeting participants accordingly.
- Schedule the meeting at a convenient date, time and location, and establish an ending time.
- When the type of meeting or number of discussion items calls for it, prepare an agenda with the topics prioritized with the more important items first. Send the agenda and any background information to participants in advance of the meeting. For meetings such as staff meetings, provide the participants an opportunity to suggest items for the agenda before it is finalized.
- The size of the meeting room should be consistent with the number of participants, and ensure that it is well ventilated and generally conducive to the conduct of a productive meeting. All audiovisual equipment should be set up in advance of the meeting.
- Designate someone, usually a junior officer, to prepare official notes of the meeting, but remember that it is also good practice for the chairperson to write down important points during the meeting with which to compare the draft minutes of record.

During the Meeting
- Begin the meeting on time. For special meetings or those held with outside attendees, delay the starting time a few minutes if some participants, especially senior officers, are not yet present.
- Introduce participants, as appropriate. State the purpose and objectives of the meeting, and announce the scheduled ending time.
- Facilitate and encourage open discussion of issues. Show interest in the discussions by posing questions and highlighting significant points. Tactfully deter those who begin to dominate the proceedings and call on other persons who might have knowledge of the subject. Show patience and impartiality in dealing with participants.

- Keep participants on track with the agenda, in terms of topics, objectives and time of the meeting. Providing a brief progress summary during a lengthy discussion is sometimes helpful. If it appears that insufficient time has been allotted to cover all agenda items, stop and discuss possible options (e.g., items that should be discussed, referred to a committee, or postponed).
- At the conclusion of the meeting, summarize the discussions and results. Recap follow-up actions to be taken, the persons responsible and time frame for completion. Thank the participants for their attendance and contributions to the meeting. If meeting minutes and/or action documents are available, distribute those within a few days to all participants.

The Participants

Meeting participants also have responsibilities that help produce a more effective meeting. Keep in mind that commissioned officers are expected to be leaders, and you can only lead by thoughtfully articulating your ideas.

Pre-Meeting
- Be prepared. Know the purpose of the meeting. If available, review the agenda and any background materials.
- If issues suggest possible conflict, prepare yourself mentally to deal with any conflict in a professional way.
- When making a presentation, experts agree that it is better to write down and present from key thoughts, rather than read from a manuscript. *(See the Section, Presentations & Speaking.)*

During the Meeting
- Be on time—it is distracting to arrive when the meeting is in progress and suggests a lack of respect, even if that is not the case.
- If you are a newcomer to a regularly held meeting, allow others to take their seats before seating yourself. Be cognizant that the organization may reserve what are termed "power" or authority positions (e.g., the head and foot of the conference table, the immediate right and left of the head position, center chairs) for senior officials.
- Be attentive and speak-up, but do not dominate a discussion. The effectiveness of a meeting is realized only when the participants maintain interest and active involvement in the discussions—stay alert and express your viewpoints. If you are bored, avoid displaying poor habits such as whispering to your neighbor, slouching in your chair, repetitious checking of your watch or doodling.

- Stay on focus. Everyone's time is valuable. If tangential issues are brought up, it is better to postpone deliberation on the matter unless there is concurrence that the new subject is pertinent and should be discussed.
- Be considerate of the thoughts and feelings of others. Because people perceive matters differently or are not versed in the nuances of all subject matters, any derision of others is generally out of place in a meeting. Do not personalize negative remarks. When on the receiving end of an unduly negative comment, do not respond in kind; keep reactive emotions under control.

Office Appointments

One-on-one and small group meetings held in an individual's office may afford the opportunity of discussing a matter in better detail, but the effectiveness of those meetings can be side tracked if a few courtesies are overlooked. Therefore, be alert to the following.

- Be on time, whether the attendee or host. If the meeting is held in your office, do not let prior meetings overrun their allotted time. If you must keep others waiting outside your office, inform them of the approximate time delay and ensure their comfort.
- For colleagues and outside attendees coming to your office, stand and welcome those attendees, offering a handshake. Introduce meeting participants to each other, including individuals' names and affiliations, and gesture to be seated. If you an attendee and no one in the host group introduces you, extend your hand to those nearby, shake hands and introduce yourself. Business cards may be exchanged at this time.
- If you are the host, offer the group refreshments and make a few, brief pleasantries, if appropriate, prior to starting discussions.
- Once the meeting has begun, do not receive telephone calls; attendees should have cell phones turned to silent mode or off. Listen attentively, ask questions and take notes. Show proper deference to senior officials (this should not, however, deter discussion of an issue). If you are leading the discussion, summarize the proceedings at the conclusion of the meeting and reiterate any agreed upon action items.
- If you are the host, thank the visiting attendees (attendees should also thank the chairperson), exchange handshakes and escort visitors out.

Conventions

Conventions include professional association meetings and other large meetings that PHS commissioned officers attend on a periodic basis. These meetings offer professional and uniformed service-related education, information and training that is often essential to remaining current on new professional practice and Commissioned Corps issues. There may also be an exhibitor area for company and government-sponsored display booths covering a myriad of products, programs and services of interest to attendees. Conventions provide a networking opportunity that is important in keeping up with acquaintances and learning about the experiences of colleagues. While there is often a social program, the importance of these meetings is primarily their program sessions. These meetings can be helpful in advancing an officer's career if a few things are kept in mind.

- As a speaker, you need to be professional in every way—thorough preparation in order to speak with authority on the seminar topic; effective presentation skills; and, high quality visuals aids (if used). *(See the Section, Presentations & Speaking.)*
- Review the agenda before each meeting day in order to select the more pertinent seminars that relate to your professional interests. Always be on time, whether the speaker or an attendee. Keep any questions you may have for the speaker brief and to the point.
- Remember that your actions during the business portion of the meeting, at receptions and after-hours are often in view by colleagues and fellow officers. Even when seminars may not be that pertinent, it is important to fulfill your responsibility to attend sessions when meeting costs are paid by your office. At other times, it is important to maintain good behavior, because your actions reflect on you *and* the USPHS.

Parliamentary Procedure

Knowledge of parliamentary procedure is essential if you are the presiding officer or are a delegate to an assembly of a large organization. The standard book on this subject is *Robert's Rules of Order Revised.* It is noteworthy that this book was originally written in 1876, with a revised edition in 1915, by General Henry M. Robert, a West Point graduate who became Chief of Engineers, U.S. Army. The book can be obtained at book stores. Following is a brief review of some basic rules.

Motions
There are different motions, classified according to their purpose, that are used to conduct the business of a meeting.

Main Motion. The main motion brings forward a new topic for consideration. A member is first recognized by the presiding officer in order to make the motion, which must be seconded by another member. When first proposed, it is a *motion,* but is thereafter referred to by the chairperson as the *question.* The chairperson restates the motion and asks if there are any remarks, at which time debate may proceed. Only one main motion may be considered at a time, and all remarks are addressed to the chairperson. A member may seek to close debate by moving *the previous question,* but all other motions having an order of precedence greater than this subsidiary motion must be dealt with first.

Subsidiary Motions. Subsidiary motions relate to a specified action on the main motion; they are used for the purpose of modifying or otherwise disposing of the main motion. The subsidiary motion must be considered before further action is taken on the main motion. Subsidiary motions yield in precedence to incidental and privileged motions. There are seven subsidiary motions, with the following precedence: lay on the table; previous question (close debate); limit or extend debate; postpone to a certain time; commit or refer (to a committee); amend; and postpone indefinitely.

Incidental Motions. Incidental motions are incident to the pending question and are dealt with as they arise. Most of these motions are not debatable. Incidental motions yield to privileged motions, but have no order of precedence among themselves. Some incidental motions are as follows: appeal from the decision of the chairperson; consider by paragraph (seriatim); division of the question; parliamentary inquiry; point of information; point of order; suspend the rules; and withdraw a motion.

Privileged Motions. Privileged motions have no direct connection to the main motion. They are used to take care of relatively urgent matters and therefore have precedence over other types of motions. There are five privileged motions, with the following precedence: fix the time at which to adjourn; adjourn; recess; raise question of privilege; and call for orders of the day.

Other Motions. There are a few other motions that have the effect of bringing a question back for consideration on the floor. These have particular rules associated with them. They include the following: take from the table; reconsider; and rescind.

Precedence of Motions
Precedence sets the priority by which motions are considered. The following list is arranged according to rank, with the highest precedence at the top of the list. Privileged and subsidiary motions have precedence within their own categories, whereas incidental motions have no order of precedence within the category. Note that the main motion is ranked last—other motions are made

while the main motion is pending, and those must be dealt with before the main motion.

Privileged Motions
By order of precedence.
Fix the time at which to adjourn
Adjourn
Take recess
Raise question of privilege
Call for orders of the day
Incidental Motions
No order of precedence.
Appeal from the decision of the chairperson*
Consider by paragraph
Division of the question
Parliamentary inquiry
Point of information
Point of order
Suspend the rules
Withdraw a motion
Subsidiary Motions
By order of precedence.
Lay on the table
Previous question (close debate)
Limit or extend debate
Postpone to a certain time*
Commit or refer (to a committee)*
Amend the amendment*
Amend the main motion*
Postpone indefinitely*
Main Motion*

* *Motions that are debatable.*

Officers are advised to refer to *Robert's Rules of Order Revised* for more detailed information.

SECTION VII.

TABLE PROTOCOL

Commissioned officers need to be familiar with proper table etiquette, because dining is something done everyday, often in the presence of colleagues. It is a generally held belief that one's dining skills reflect upbringing. While table etiquette obviously has minimal importance on the battlefield, in business, as the term is broadly applied, ability at the dining table influences the perception of others with respect to a person's professional competence and the organization they represent.

> TABLE SETTINGS
> TABLE MANNERS
> RESTAURANT DINING

Table Settings

All officers should be familiar with the placement and use of dining utensils, china and crystal. Such knowledge, combined with good table manners, is considered basic to an officer's social abilities.

To begin, a formal multicourse place setting is depicted in Figure 1. Less formal place settings follow the same pattern, but with fewer items than are shown in the figure. The formality of the occasion will guide the selection of the type, quality, color and proper usage of flatware, china, crystal, condiment servers, napkins, tablecloth, centerpiece and candles. At a formal dinner, flatware should be silverplate or sterling.

Flatware
Placement. Flatware is set with the handle ends about one inch from the edge of the table. It is placed on both sides of, and optionally above, the main plate, with forks placed to the left, and knives and spoons to the right. The utensils are arranged in order of use from the outside in, corresponding to the courses of

the meal. For example, a salad fork may be located on either side of the dinner fork, depending on when the salad is to be served (i.e., before or, in the European manner, after the main course). The dessert fork and spoon may be placed above the main plate, as in Figure 1, placed in the inside positions of the forks and spoons or brought to the table when dessert is served.

Figure 1. Formal Place Setting

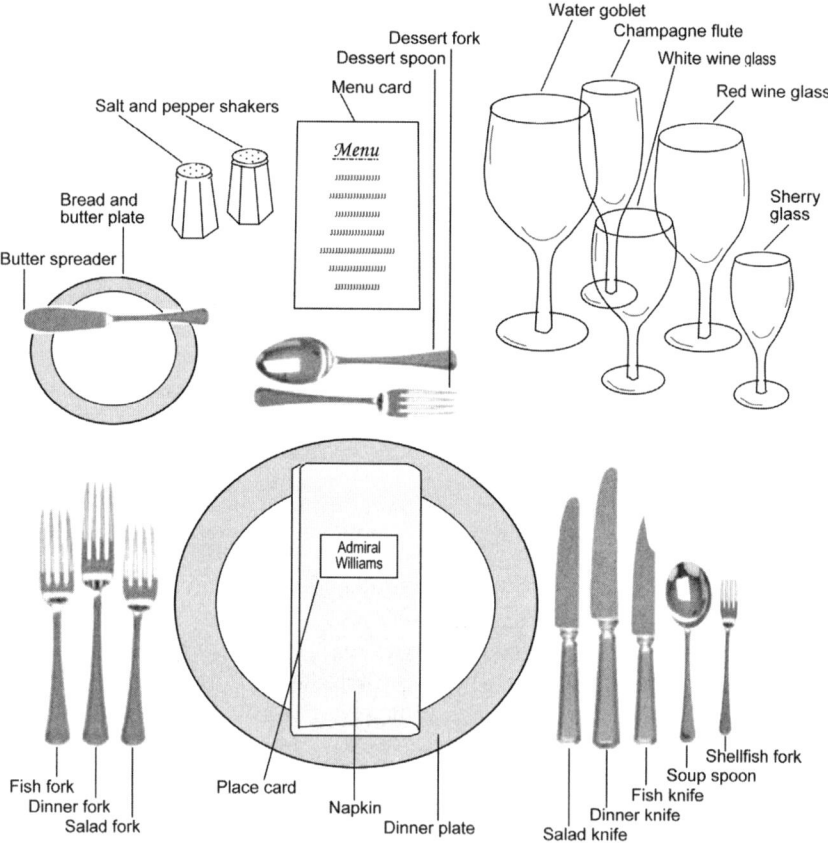

With the exception of the addition of an oyster/shellfish fork placed to the right of the spoon(s), there are never more than three forks and/or three knives in the place setting. If another fork or knife is needed, it is placed on the table when the course is served. Note that knife blades always face toward the plate.

The soup spoon, which may be round (clear soup) or more oval (cream soup) is placed to the right of the knives.

The butter knife or spreader is placed straight, or at a slight diagonal from upper left to lower right, across the top rim of the butter plate, with the blade facing inward.

A demitasse spoon or teaspoon is placed to the right of the coffee cup and saucer when it is served. Though properly served after the dessert course, coffee is often served with dessert.

Use. Soup should be spooned away from you, inside the bowl. Sip the soup from the side of the spoon (i.e., not from the tip). Used spoons are placed on the saucer or underplate of the dish, or may be placed in the bowl if it is shallow.

There are two methods for handling a fork and knife, referred to as the American and Continental styles—both styles are acceptable in the U.S., with the Continental style becoming more prevalent.

In both styles, the fork is held in your left hand, tines pointing down, to hold the food in place, and the knife is held in your right hand to cut it. In the *American style,* the knife is returned to the plate and the fork is transferred to the right hand, tines up, to pick up the piece of food. In the *Continental style,* the fork remains in the left hand and, with tines still down, the piece of food is conveyed by fork to your mouth; the knife remains in your right hand as long as needed.

Figure 2. Holding the Fork

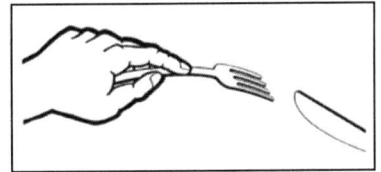

Whichever style is used, when the fork is in the left hand with tines pointing down, the index finger extends over the shaft (Figure 2). The fork handle should *not* be held as if it were a pencil, nor gripped in the palm of your hand at a 90° angle to the dinner plate.

When not in use, a knife is placed diagonally across the upper right edge of the plate, blade facing the center of the plate.

When you are not finished eating and want to pause, leave the knife diagonally across the upper right edge of the plate and place the fork in a parallel position, tines up and centered on the plate. Alternatively, use the European style, crossing the fork, tines down, handle lower left, and the knife, handle lower right, in the center of the plate.

Figure 3. Finished Position

When finished eating, the fork and knife are customarily placed together across the middle of the plate, horizontally from right to left or diagonally from lower right to upper left, with the knife above the fork, blade turned inward, and fork tines up or down (Figure 3).

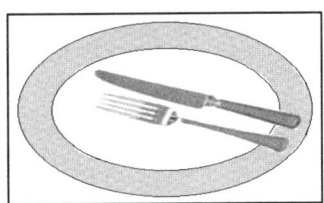

China

Placement. The place setting can include a service plate (also referred to as a charger or place plate), upon which may be placed the pre-entrée dishes or salad plate. The service plate or dinner plate is at the center of the place setting, with all other place setting items arranged around it (Figure 1).

At a formal dinner, a salad plate will not be on the table when there is a separate salad course, in which case the salad plate is placed in the main plate area when it is served.

Use. Dishes used for the appetizer, soup and/or dessert may be placed upon the service plate, if present. When there is no salad plate and/or butter plate, the dinner plate is used for salad and butter. A bread/roll can be placed on the dinner plate, or, on the tablecloth if it is *un*buttered. A bowl should be tipped away from you to spoon out residual liquid.

Serving dishes are passed around the table to the right (counterclockwise). When passing a dish to another person, hold the serving dish so that a handle of the dish, and serving utensil(s) if present, are readily available for the other diner to grasp.

Crystal

Placement. Glassware is located above and toward the right of the dinner plate. Crystal may consist of the water goblet or tumbler, plus other glasses depending on the dinner courses to be served. Other glasses may include, from right to left: a sherry glass (sherry is consumed with certain soups); wine glass (it two are present, one is for white wine which is typically consumed with a fish course or, absent the sherry glass, sometimes with soup; the other wine glass is for red wine); and, champagne glass (for the entire dinner or dessert, and toasting).

Use. A water goblet or other large stem glass is held at the base of its bowl, and a tumbler near its base. A wine glass should be held by its stem to keep the glass unsmudged and, if applicable, help chilled wines remain cool. Your mouth should be empty and lips clean before drinking from crystal to avoid leaving food particles on the rim.

Condiment Servers

Placement. Condiments should be transferred from their package containers to serving dishes. There should be a salt and pepper set for every one to three diners. Occasionally, salt cellars or pepper pots (small open bowls with spoons), or pepper mills are provided instead of shakers.

Use. Depending on the formality of the meal, condiments will either be offered by a waiter or placed on the table. A small amount of each condiment is placed on your butter or dinner plate, as appropriate, and not directly on the food for which it is intended.

Napkins

Placement. Cloth napkins, either matched or color coordinated with the table cloth or place mats, should be used. They are usually folded into a rectangle (by folding in half or thirds in each direction to form a square, then folding the two sides, each equal to one-third of the width, over or under) or chevron style (by folding as above into a square, then diagonally in half, and then tucking the pointed ends under). Napkins are placed on the table in the main plate area or on the service plate if one is utilized. If the first course, such as appetizer or soup, is in place when diners arrive at the table, the napkin is located to the left of the forks. If a monogram is on the napkin, it should be visible.

Use. Upon being seated at a table, unfold the napkin as much as needed and place it on your lap; if the dinner is hosted, wait until after the host has begun to put a napkin on his/her lap. In using the napkin, the mouth should be patted or only lightly wiped. At the end of the meal, the napkin is neatly gathered (*not* re-folded to its original shape) and placed on the table to the left of the place setting, or in the center if plates have been removed.

Place Cards/Menu Cards

At larger functions or when guest ranking is needed, place cards may be used to indicate where individuals are to be seated. Place cards and menu cards are normally white or cream color, with or without a gold or silver border. They can be handwritten, typed or printed and, at a uniformed service event, lettering is in black ink.

Place Cards. Place cards are up to 3½" wide by 2" high, and are laid flat on the table above the place setting, or on the folded napkin on the service plate. Folded place cards are up to 3" high after folding in half, and are placed on the table above the service plate. For more formal occasions, only an officer's rank and surname are written. If two officers have the same last name, their full names are written on the cards.

Menu Cards. Menu cards are up to 5" wide by 7" high. They are set on the table or upright in a holder, centered above each place setting; or, they may be leaned against the glassware, placed on the folded napkin on the service plate or set on the table between every two diners.

Centerpiece and Candles

A centerpiece comprised of flowers or other decorative arrangement is placed at the middle of the table. The centerpiece should be low enough or very thin (e.g., tall clear glass vase) to permit diners to see each other across the table. If candlesticks are used, one or a pair of candlesticks or a candelabrum is placed at the midpoints between the centerpiece and each end of the table. Candles are normally white or, at less formal occasions, color coordinated with the table linens; they should be of sufficient height that the flame will stay above eye level. The candles are lighted prior to seating diners, and should remain lit until guests have departed from the dining area. Candlesticks (in contrast to small or votive candles) are not appropriate for the luncheon table but, if present, should be for decorative purposes only and not lit.

Seating Arrangements
For a formal dinner hosted by husband and wife, the host and hostess sit at opposite ends of the table. If female and male guests are equal in number, seating is alternated female-male along the table, noting that spouses are usually not seated beside each other. Consideration should also be given to seating a left-handed guest at a left corner, in order to prevent elbow bumping with the person to his left.

Occasionally, the purpose of the function or the stature of table guests warrants ranked seating. When ranking of guests is involved, seating is begun with the female guest of honor and next most important female to the host's right and left, respectively; and the male guest of honor and next most important male to the hostess' right and left, respectively. See also the Section, *Official Dinners & Receptions*.

Table Manners

Table manners are commonly felt to be a reflection of one's upbringing and have a significant impact on how others perceive you professionally, as well as socially. Table manners should be learned to the extent that they become a natural part of one's behavior, without having to think of the "rules." This section should be reviewed along with the Sections, *Table Settings* and *Restaurant Dining*.

Before the Meal
Whether a business luncheon or professional meeting banquet, certain protocol should be followed. Upon being seated at the table, the napkin should be unfolded (large napkins may remain half folded) and placed on your lap, with two provisos: if the meal is hosted, wait until after the host has begun to place a napkin on his/her lap; and, if it is known that an invocation is to be said within a few minutes, your napkin should not be unfolded beforehand. Other than placing the napkin on your lap and taking a sip of water or other beverage, nothing on the table should be disturbed while waiting.

As others arrive at the table, those already seated should stand for face-to-face introductions. Absent such introductions, men need not stand when business, professional or military women colleagues join the table. However, as a courtesy, junior officers should rise when a flag officer joins the table.

You should sit in the chair with back posture comfortably erect. When at the table, do not fidget (e.g., drumming the table with your fingers, touching or combing your hair). While waiting for the meal, in between courses and after the meal, your hands may rest in your lap, hands (at the wrists) may rest on the table edge, or elbows/forearms may rest near the table edge.

If an item (flatware, china, crystal, napkin) is missing from the place service, ask for the item. If an item is unclean, ask for a replacement—do not clean it yourself.

Service of the Meal

Before or after guests are seated, water glasses are filled. When a server is present, courses are placed in front of you by the server from the left side. Except for items on your extreme left, dinnerware is removed from the right side when the course is finished. When platters of food are offered by the server, guests should use both the serving fork and spoon to transfer a moderate portion of food to their plates; if a piece of toast is underneath, it is transferred with the food. Also take a portion of any vegetables and garnishes which accompany an entrée on the platter.

At a hosted dinner where a server is not present, food service begins with the person to the host's right and proceeds in that direction (counterclockwise) around the table to the host, who is served last. Diners also pass serving dishes of food and condiments around the table to the right. When an item on the table is out of reach, ask the person nearest the item to "Please pass the (item)." Salt and pepper shakers are passed as a set, even when only one of them is requested. Place a condiment next to, and not on, the food it is to accompany; gravy and fluid sauces, however, are placed directly on the meat. Foods such as celery and radishes are placed on the butter plate, if present. Bread or rolls will usually be served when the soup or an initial course of salad is served. Where there is no butter plate, an unbuttered bread or roll may be placed on the tablecloth. Although a salad course may be served after the main course, it is more typically served before or with the entrée. If not already on the main course plate or in a small dish near the dinner plate, the server will offer vegetables to each guest from a serving dish. Coffee or tea may be served with the meal, but is more correctly served with, or after, the dessert.

When there is foreign material such as hair or a small insect in food, the material should, it not too unsettling, be removed and the food eaten at a dinner hosted in the home; otherwise, inform the host. In a restaurant, bring it to the server's attention and have the dish replaced.

Wine Service

Wine may be identified as apéritif (appetizer) wines, dinner wines, and after-dinner/dessert wines. Apéritif wines are generally fortified and commonly include the dry sherries and vermouths, or they may be sparkling wines. For the main course, a dry white wine is typically served with fish, a white or light red (blush or rosé) wine is served with poultry and white meat (e.g., pork), and a red wine with wild fowl and red meat. However, it is acceptable to have white, blush or red wine with any food, and serve only one wine, including champagne, as the dinner wine. Dessert wines are generally sweeter and most are fortified, and include sweet sherries, ports, sauternes and sweet champagnes.

White and blush/rosé wines should be served slightly chilled (about $50°$ F.), red wines at room temperature (about $70°$ F.), and sparkling wines well chilled. White wines are opened just before use, whereas red wines should be uncorked one-half to one hour before the meal to permit development of its bouquet.

White wine may be served prior to a first course; otherwise, wine is served when food is brought to the table. The wine will be presented to the host or person who ordered it to review the label to ensure it is the correct wine and vintage. The waiter will remove and place the bottle cork on the table for the host to examine—it should not be dried out. A small amount of wine is then poured into the host's wine glass, who may tip the glass slightly to look for bright color and clarity. He should gently swirl the wine in the glass to release its aroma, sniff and then take a sip of wine to make sure it is alright (has not soured). If satisfactory, he nods approval to the server. If the wine is served at a dinner in the home, the host should check the wine *before* it is brought to the table. The server will pour the wine into each diner's wine glass, about half full, beginning with the person to the host's right and continuing counterclockwise around the table until the host is served.

During the Meal
In smaller groups, begin eating only after everyone has been served and, if applicable, the host starts. In larger groups, you may proceed after several guests have been served and it is evident that service will be uneven; if a hosted function, the host should indicate to those already served to begin.

Whether eating American or Continental style, only one or two pieces of food are cut at a time for consumption. Food should be brought to your mouth, such that there is minimal bending of your body to meet the fork or spoon. In certain instances, foods such as asparagus (not juicy or covered with sauce), bacon (crisp), celery, chicken (informal meal) and sandwiches may be picked up with the fingers. However, if in doubt about whether to use your fingers, even when it is otherwise proper, always opt for using a utensil, particularly at a business meal, formal dinner or an official function.
You should chew food with your mouth closed, and talk only when your mouth is not full.
- If an uncut loaf of bread is served, the host (if present) should cut several slices before it is passed on to guests.
- For bread and rolls, break off a small piece to be consumed and, holding it near the butter plate, butter that portion. Hot breads such as muffins and rolls are cut in half and may be entirely buttered before eating; toast should be buttered first, and then cut in half.
- All edible garnishes (such as cherries, orange slices, parsley, watercress) that are served with beverages and food may be eaten.

- Vegetables which are served in a side dish may be eaten with a fork directly from the dish or transferred with your fork or spoon to the dinner plate.

Remove troublesome food, bones or pits from your mouth with as little notice as possible, by expelling the item onto a spoon or fork or by grasping it with your thumb and index finger; place the item on your plate and cover it with a bit of food, if necessary. If food gets lodged in your teeth, excuse yourself from the table and dislodge it in the restroom or wait until the meal is completed; do not use a toothpick or your finger to dislodge food at the table (this is in contrast to etiquette in some Asian countries). Never lick your fingers after using your hands to eat; use your napkin.

While eating, the hand/wrist not in use may be rested in your lap or on the table edge, but one's elbows should not be on the table. Cover your mouth with the napkin to burp, and then quietly say "Excuse me." If about to cough or sneeze, cover your mouth and nose with your handkerchief (if readily available) or napkin. Use only a handkerchief or tissue to blow your nose; if necessary, excuse yourself from the table. A woman may quickly check her make-up at the table, but neither women nor men should comb or otherwise touch their hair at the dining table.

Small beverage spills may be removed from clothing or tablecloth by blotting with your napkin. Food spills may be removed with a clean piece of flatware, as well. For spills that require a damp cloth, excuse yourself and go the restroom.

Flatware that has been picked up and used should not be placed on the table again. The principal utensils are placed on the main plate and, for example, spoons used for soup are placed in a shallow bowl or on the soup bowl underplate, and spoons used to stir coffee or iced tea are placed on the edge of the saucer. Note that any *unused* flatware should be left in place on the table and not put with the used utensils.

Before dessert is served, the table is cleared of serving dishes, dinnerware and condiments, and the table is crumbed (i.e., the bread crumbs are removed). At a business meal or formal dinner, diners should not hand plates to the server unless it is very evident that a particular item on the table cannot be reached.

Occasionally, finger bowls are offered before or after dessert. Normally, the finger bowl with a doily underneath is placed on the dessert plate, with the dessert fork and spoon to each side of the bowl. Dip the fingers of each hand into the bowl and dry them with your napkin. Then, remove the dessert fork and spoon from the plate and place them to the left and right side of the plate, respectively. With both hands, move the finger bowl and doily to a position at the upper left of your place setting.

Toasts

A toast is offered to honor individuals or institutions and imparts a special significance to an event. The host, a senior officer or the official who organized a dinner should make the first toast. This is typically done once the dessert has been served and wine or champagne glasses are filled. See the Sections, *Dining-In & Dining-Out* and *Official Dinners & Receptions* for detailed information.

Restaurant Dining

Restaurant dining, when other than a routine lunch with colleagues, may be for the purpose of conducting business, marking an organization-related occasion, or may be primarily social in nature. Whatever the purpose, restaurant dining requires a familiarity with some protocol that is in addition to general table etiquette. This section should be reviewed along with the Sections, *Table Settings* and *Table Manners*.

Reservations

If you are hosting a lunch or dinner in a restaurant, you will be responsible for arrangements and coordination of the meal. Planning ahead, particularly for larger groups, is often essential to ensure a successful event. Select the restaurant based on the desired ambience for the function, preferences (if known) of guests and convenience of location. When telephoning the restaurant to make the reservation, you should specify any special requirements or service you want, such as requesting a more secluded area of the restaurant, or requesting a certain method for paying the bill.

For very important occasions, visit the restaurant beforehand and confirm all arrangements, including, if applicable, where individuals are to sit. You should also consider providing the maître d' (headwaiter) with a tip in advance of the function.

Arrival and Seating

The host should be at the restaurant early enough to greet arriving guests. Upon arrival, guests should check overcoats and umbrellas at the checkroom. Telephone the restaurant when you know that you will be quite late. If the host or some guests have not arrived on time, the maître d' should be so informed by those present. They usually then have the option of staying at the restaurant's waiting area or proceeding to the table to wait for the others to arrive.

Nothing on the dining table should be disturbed while waiting for others. If, however, ten to fifteen minutes have elapsed and everyone is still not present, begin with any drink orders. It is generally recommended that a person limit oneself to one or at most two cocktails or glasses of wine before the meal. "Nondrinkers" should consider ordering a nonalcoholic beverage. If someone you know is seated elsewhere in the restaurant, avoid leaving the table, but merely nod in acknowledgement to the other person when eye contact is made.

As guests arrive at the table, the host should stand, greet and introduce them, as appropriate. As a courtesy, junior officers should also stand when very senior officers arrive at the table. The best seats, such as armchairs, seats which are away from busy aisles or the banquette (bench seat along a wall) should be given to senior officers and visiting guests. If you need the undivided attention of others to discuss business, consider requesting a table in a secluded part of the restaurant. If seating is prearranged, men and women should be dispersed around the table, such that there is no apparent segregation. At larger functions where there is an honored guest, he/she is seated to the right of the host.

Ordering

Food. The host should recommend a few items on the menu for which the restaurant is noted and suggest, if budget is not a concern, one or two expensive main courses to signal to guests that they should feel free to order what they want. Otherwise, guests should select a moderately priced menu item (in other words, select neither the least nor most expensive item, because either might be a slight to the host). Items are ordered à la carte, where each item is separately priced, or table d'hôte, a complete meal at a set price. Guests should not hesitate to ask the waiter about specialty dishes or for his recommendation. On the other hand, it is unwise at more official lunches or dinners to ask the waiter about a dish you should ordinarily know about or when you are unsure how to pronounce it. When the primary function of the meal is to conduct business, ease of consumption should also be kept in mind when selecting the main course. Each person should order for himself and be ready to answer the waiter's inquiries about selections and food preparation.

Wine. After all food orders are taken, the host should order wine, if it is desired. The wine order will be taken by the waiter or a wine steward (sommelier). The host who has little knowledge of wines should either ask the waiter/wine steward for his recommendation or ask a knowledgeable guest to make the selection. A good quality wine should be chosen, based on what most people have selected for their main course. White and red wines may both be ordered, although a carefully chosen white or red wine only will often complement any combination of foods.

Conversation

If the function is a business meal, the host should initiate the business discussion. Conversation should be limited to small talk until the waiter has taken everyone's order, including the wine order, and removed the menus; only then should business discussions commence. If the function is more social in nature, each guest has some responsibility to ensure that his neighbors at the table are included in conversation. For example, after conversing for a while with the person to his right, a diner should turn to the neighbor on his left and initiate a dialogue.

Eating

Eating should begin only after everyone has been served, unless it is apparent that the service is unduly delayed and to wait would result in the meals already served becoming cold. If there is a guest of honor, he should begin eating first, followed by the other guests and then the host. Absent an honored guest, the host should urge everyone to begin if there is hesitation.

In addition to the information contained in the Sections, *Table Settings* and *Table Manners*, there are several things to note when eating in a restaurant.

- It is the host's responsibility to manage the table and call a waiter to the table when needed. Guests should keep complaints to a minimum and quietly convey any problems to the host or, at larger affairs or absent a host, to the waiter.
- When coffee cups are turned upside down on their saucers, turn them upright when coffee is being poured to receive coffee service.
- Empty unit-of-use condiment containers or packets should be put on an unused plate. If a plate is not available, butter, jelly or marmalade containers may be placed on, or next to, the butter plate; empty sugar packets should be folded and placed on, under or next to the rim of the coffee cup saucer or butter plate.
- Call the waiter to replace unclean or dropped utensils (do not wipe them off with your napkin) and to clean up spills on the floor.
- Requesting a "doggie bag" at the end of a meal may be acceptable on certain social dining occasions where guests are well known to each other; it is inappropriate, however, when dining with professional associates.

Receiving the Bill

Upon receiving the check, the host should quickly review it for accuracy and then pay in cash, by credit or debit card, or sign for the check if he has an account at the restaurant. Alternatively, the host may prefer to accept the check away from the table, or he may sign the credit card charge slip in advance of the function and request that the receipt be sent to him—such arrangements should be confirmed with the waiter beforehand.

Social Receptions

Social receptions offer a means to renew professional relationships and to meet and socialize with many people at one place and time. Occasions where alcoholic beverages are served as a primary part of the function include the cocktail party, cocktail-buffet party, the pre-dinner drink hour, and receptions.

The societal trend toward a reduction in the consumption of alcoholic drinks had led to sponsors offering a wider selection of nonalcoholic beverages for guests. In all cases, there are some general considerations to keep in mind.

Considerations for the Host

Plan Well. There are a number of things to consider in planning a social.
- Telephone or send written invitations at least two to three weeks in advance of a party. The beginning and ending time of the function should be specified. For the sake of efficiency, the R.S.V.P. on written invitations may state "Regrets Only" with a telephone number.
- The room for the function should be large enough for guests to easily wander about without jostling each other. The room must be well ventilated.
- Ensure a reasonably well stocked liquor selection and a variety of low calorie and nonalcoholic beverages. Ice and garnishes should be in plentiful supply.
- At a cocktail function in the home, ensure a sufficient quantity of glasses (e.g., highball, on-the-rocks, wine glasses), napkins, coasters, and a few strategically placed bar trays for used glasses and napkins.
- At larger functions, office staff should be available to assist with beverage and food service, and to facilitate guest introductions and conviviality.

Greeting Guests. Unless the function is a large convention-type reception, guests should be greeted upon arrival and helped with any coats, hats and umbrellas. They should be briefed on the layout of bars and food tables, and introduced to other guests who are present.

Handling Difficult Guests. Unwelcome hangers-on after the social has ended and guests who are inebriated should be dealt with firmly, but with tact and kindness. The host is normally responsible for the safety of guests, and anyone who appears to be functionally impaired must be assisted in whatever way necessary to ensure that the person is safely returned to his/her home or hotel. If necessary, overnight accommodations should be arranged for the person.

Considerations for the Guest

Be on Time. It is important to be on time. For cocktail parties and receptions, arrival should be no later than 15 to 30 minutes after the starting time. Normally, for pre-dinner drinks, cocktail-buffets and primarily business functions, one should arrive within 15 minutes of the scheduled starting time.

Badges. At large receptions, guests may be given name badges. Badges should be placed on the right coat lapel or area of clothing which covers the right upper chest—in this position, people can most easily glance at one another's badge when they meet and shake hands.

Consuming Beverages. Always use a cocktail napkin with iced drinks to contain drips and to avoid presenting a cold, wet hand in a handshake. Most importantly, consume alcoholic drinks conservatively. It is very difficult to regain a reputation for stability and being in control when your conversation or behavior has publicly deteriorated due to alcohol intake. For particularly long receptions, it may be advisable to decide on a specific limit to the number of alcoholic drinks consumed, and then one should sip drinks slowly and alternate with nonalcoholic drinks. Do not linger around the immediate bar area after receiving your drink.

Consuming Food. Whatever the type of function, do not overindulge. Avoid standing near the hors d'oeuvres or buffet table for long periods of time, so you do not give the appearance of being wedded to the food and to allow easy access to the table by other guests.

Conversation. Topics of discussion at a cocktail function should generally be light. Unless a business function, office matters should be avoided, especially in the presence of a senior officer, unless that person initiates the subject. Give full attention to the person with whom you are talking; avoid the "glazed" eye look or allowing your eyes to wander. Do not unload particularly personal information that could make you or the listener uneasy when back in the office.

Follow-up. If, after accepting an invitation to a function, you are unable to attend, you should telephone the host as soon as is possible. If you are unexpectedly unable to attend at the time of the function, contact the host immediately (if appropriate) or the next day with an apology and a brief explanation for your absence. After attending a function, particularly when hosted by a colleague, it is a good idea to send a thank you note.

SECTION VIII.
U.S. PUBLIC HEALTH SERVICE

There are seven uniformed services of the United States: the Public Health Service, Air Force, Army, Coast Guard, Marine Corps, National Oceanic and Atmospheric Administration, and Navy. Each of the uniformed services has certain characteristics that identify it as a unique service organization. The U.S. Public Health Service has a proud history of serving the public health needs of the Nation, and its reach now extends internationally. While acknowledging its 200-year heritage, the PHS is forging ahead in ways that will herald a new era in its history.

> MISSION
> ORGANIZATION
> OFFICE OF THE SURGEON GENERAL
> AGENCY ASSIGNMENTS
> REGULAR CORPS
> PHS HISTORY
> PHS FLAG
> PHS SEAL
> PHS CC SEAL
> PHS MARCH
> PHS COIN

Mission

The official mission of the Public Health Service (PHS) Commissioned Corps is "Protecting, promoting, and advancing the health and safety of the Nation." The Commissioned Corps achieves this mission through rapid and effective response to public health needs, leadership and excellence in public health practices, and the advancement of public health science.

The PHS Commissioned Corps is comprised of highly-trained health professionals who carry out health-related programs, understand and prevent disease and injury, assure safe and effective drugs and medical devices, deliver health services to Federal beneficiaries, and furnish health expertise in time of war or other national or international emergencies. These health professionals may be assigned to Federal, state or local agencies or international organizations to accomplish the PHS mission. To accomplish this mission, the agencies/programs are designed to:

- Help provide healthcare and related services to medically underserved populations and to other population groups with special needs.
- Prevent and control disease, identify health hazards in the environment and help correct them, and promote healthy lifestyles for the Nation's citizens.
- Improve the Nation's mental health.
- Ensure that drugs and medical devices are safe and effective, food is safe and wholesome, cosmetics are harmless, and that electronic products do not expose users to dangerous amounts of radiation.
- Conduct and support biomedical, behavioral, and health services research and communicate research results to health professionals and the public.
- Work with other nations and international agencies on global health problems and their solutions.

Organization

The Public Health Service is a principal component of the Department of Health and Human Services (HHS). It consists of the Office of Public Health and Science (headed by the Assistant Secretary for Health, and including the Office of the Surgeon General); eight operating divisions or agencies; and ten Regional Health Administrators. The Office of the Surgeon General is led by the U.S. Surgeon General, who is appointed by the President with the advice and consent of the Senate for a four-year term of office. The U.S. Surgeon General holds the rank of Vice Admiral.

The PHS Commissioned Corps has over 6,000 officers in the following professional categories: dentist, dietitian, engineer, environmental health, health services, nurse, pharmacist, physician, scientist, therapist, and veterinarian. Officers are deployed throughout the world, and are assigned to agencies within HHS and other Federal and state entities; for example, PHS officers provide health care services to members of the U.S. Coast Guard. In times of war, PHS officers may be assigned to any of the armed forces, as necessary. Since its earliest days, the Corps has provided the Public Health Service with a centrally-administered, flexible, mobile and highly trained cadre of health professionals who have served with distinction in a wide variety of clinical, research and public health leadership positions.

Office of the Surgeon General (OSG)
There are five components of the Office of the Surgeon General.
- *Immediate Office of the Surgeon General (IOSG)*
  The IOSG supports the activities and priorities of the Surgeon General, advises the HHS Assistant Secretary for Health (ASH) on matters relating to protecting and advancing the public health of the Nation; implements policies, manages and supervises the operations of the PHS Commissioned Corps; and serves as spokesperson and represents the HHS. Included within the IOSG is the Office of Military Liaison and Veteran Affairs.
- *Office of Commissioned Corps Operations (OCCO)*
  OCCO provides advice to the SG, and implements policies relating to the daily operation of the Commissioned Corps; manages personnel activities that include officer appointment, promotion, assimilation, award recognition, performance evaluation, recruitment, training, preparation of orders, and retirement. Within OCCO are four Divisions.
  - Division of Commissioned Corps Assignment
  - Division of Commissioned Corps Officer Support
  - Division of Commissioned Corps Recruitment
  - Division of Commissioned Corps Training and Career Development
- *Office of Force Readiness and Deployment (OFRD)*
  OFRD directs the mobilization and deployment of Corps officers during emergency activations, and administers readiness and response activities to include maintenance of deployment systems and conducting mission critical training. The OFRD also includes the Medical Reserve Corps (MRC) program, a specialized component of the USA Freedom Corps. The MRC program serves as a clearinghouse for information and best practices to help communities establish, implement and maintain MRC units across the Nation.
- *Office of Reserve Affairs (ORA)*
  ORA maintains Reserve components or assets, and coordinates the assignments of Corps reserve personnel.
- *Office of Science and Communications (OSC)*
  OSC advises the Surgeon General on public health issues and priorities; coordinates activities in the development of authoritative reports; prepares correspondence, speeches and communications for the SG; and represents the SG at conferences.

Office of Public Health and Science (OPHS)
The OPHS is headed by the Assistant Secretary for Health who, in concert with the Surgeon General, determines policy for the Commissioned Corps. Within the OPHS are the OSG, and the Office of Commissioned Corps Force Management which provides advice and consultation to the ASH and OSG relating to administration and oversight of the PHS Commissioned Corps.

- **Office of Commissioned Corps Force Management (OCCFM)**
  OCCFM develops policies and carries out a comprehensive force management program for the Commissioned Corps, including preparing workforce and officer standards, and overseeing the Commissioned Corps personnel services budget.

Office of the Surgeon General

The Office of the Surgeon General (OSG), under the direction of the Surgeon General, oversees the Commissioned Corps of the U.S. Public Health Service and provides support for the Surgeon General in the accomplishment of his/her other duties.

Responsibilities
In carrying out all responsibilities, the Surgeon General reports to the Assistant Secretary for Health (ASH), who is a principal advisor to the Secretary of Health and Human Services on public health and scientific issues. The Surgeon General is tasked with a myriad of responsibilities related to ensuring the health and welfare of the Nation. He/she commands the Commissioned Corps, including managing the Corps' operations, force readiness and field deployments. Among his other duties are to issue warnings to the public on identified health hazards; maintain ongoing communication with professional groups; represent the PHS at national and international public health and professional meetings; provide management and oversight of the Medical Reserve Corps program; and provide liaison with governmental and private organizations on matters pertaining to military and veterans affairs.

History
In 1798, Congress established the U.S. Marine Hospital Service—predecessor of today's U.S. Public Health Service—to provide health care to sick and injured merchant seamen. In 1870, the Marine Hospital Service was reorganized as a national hospital system with centralized administration under a medical officer, the Supervising Surgeon, who was later given the title of Surgeon General.

Dr. John Woodworth, appointed as the first Supervising Surgeon in 1871, established a cadre of medical personnel to administer the Marine Hospital System. In 1889, the Congress recognized this new personnel system by formally authorizing the Commissioned Corps. At first only open to physicians, over the years the Corps' responsibilities have expanded, to include a commensurate broad range of health professionals.

Prior to 1968, the Surgeon General was the head of the PHS, and all program, administrative, and financial management authorities flowed through the Surgeon General, who reported directly to the Secretary of Health, Education, and Welfare (predecessor of HHS). In 1968, pursuant to a reorganization plan issued by the President, the Secretary delegated line responsibility for the PHS to the Assistant Secretary for Health. Between 1972 and 1981, various organizational configurations were in place; for example, from 1977 until 1981, the positions of Assistant Secretary for Health and the Surgeon General were combined. However, in 1987, the OSG was reestablished as a staff office within the OASH. Concomitant with this action, the Surgeon General again became responsible for management of the Commissioned Corps personnel system.

In 1987, Surgeon General C. Everett Koop launched a major effort to revitalize the Corps. Actions were taken to enhance all aspects of Corps management, and to make sure that agencies utilizing officers are actively involved in the formulation and review of PHS policies.

In 2002, the Commissioned Corps began a new phase in Corps history known as the Transformation of the Corps. Surgeon General Richard Carmona leads the Corps as it undertakes this comprehensive transformation to better prepare it to protect, promote and advance the health and safety of the Nation.

Surgeons General
The first Supervising Surgeon of the Marine Hospital Service was appointed in 1871. That position became supervising Surgeon General in 1873, and Surgeon General in 1902. As of 2005, with the incumbent Surgeon General Richard H. Carmona, there have been seventeen individuals who have served in this position.

> **Surgeon General**
> John M. Woodworth, 1871 – 1879
> John B. Hamilton, 1879 – 1891
> Walter Wyman, 1891 – 1911
> Rupert Blue, 1912 – 1920
> Hugh S. Cumming, 1920 – 1936
> Thomas Parran, Jr., 1936 – 1948
> Leonard A. Scheele, 1948 – 1956
> Leroy E. Burney, 1956 – 1961
> Luther L. Terry, 1961 – 1965
> William H. Stewart, 1965 – 1969
> Jesse L. Steinfeld, 1969 – 1973
> Julius B. Richmond, 1977 – 1981
> C. Everett Koop, 1981 – 1989
> Antonia C. Novello, 1990 – 1993
> M. Joycelyn Elders, 1993 – 1994
> David Satcher, 1998 – 2002
> Richard H. Carmona (Incumbent), 2002 – Present

In addition, the following individuals served as Acting Surgeon General:
S. Paul Ehrlich (Acting), 1972 – 1977
Audrey F. Manley (Acting), 1995 – 1997
J. Jarrett Clinton (Acting), 1997 – 1998
Kenneth P. Moritsugu (Acting), 2002

Deputy Surgeons General
The Deputy Surgeon General (DSG) has a critical role within the OSG. Particularly in the last few decades, the DSG has been an active partner with the Surgeon General in the development of new policy with respect to the revitalization and transformation of the Commissioned Corps. The DSG is responsible for overseeing the daily operations of the Commissioned Corps and serving in the place of the SG, as needed. The following individuals have served in the DSG position:

Deputy Surgeon General
Warren F. Draper, 1944 – 1946
James A. Crabtree, 1946 – 1948
W. Palmer Dearing, 1948 – 1957
John D. Porterfield, 1957 – 1962
David Price, 1962 – 1965
Leo Gehrig, 1965 – 1968
S. Paul Ehrlich, 1968 – 1977
John C. Greene, 1978 – 1981
Faye G. Abdellah, 1981 – 1989
O. Marie Henry, 1990 – 1992
Robert A. Whitney, 1992 – 1993
Audrey F. Manley, 1994 – 1997
Kenneth P. Moritsugu (Incumbent), 1998 – Present

Agency Assignments

The USPHS Commissioned Corps, unlike other uniformed services, does not directly employ its officers, with the exception of those who administer the commissioned personnel program. PHS officers are assigned to HHS and certain non-HHS Federal agencies and programs. The following is a brief description of agencies, operating divisions (OpDivs) and programs where commissioned officers may serve.

Agencies within HHS
to which PHS Officers are Assigned
(Often referred to as Operating Divisions)

Agency for Healthcare Research and Quality (AHRQ)
AHRQ supports research designed to improve the outcomes and quality of healthcare, reduce its costs, address patient safety and medical errors, and broaden access to effective services. The research sponsored, conducted and disseminated by AHRQ provides information that helps people make better decisions about healthcare.

Agency for Toxic Substances and Disease Registry (ATSDR)
ATSDR's mission is to prevent exposure and adverse human health effects and diminished quality of life associated with exposure to hazardous substances from waste sites, unplanned release and other sources of pollution present in the environment.

Centers for Disease Control and Prevention (CDC)
CDC's mission is to promote health and quality of life by preventing and controlling disease, injury, and disability. CDC seeks to accomplish this mission by working with partners throughout the Nation and world to monitor health, detect and investigate health problems, conduct research to enhance prevention, develop and advocate sound public health policies, implement prevention strategies, promote healthy behaviors, foster safe and healthful environments, and provide leadership and training.

Food and Drug Administration (FDA)
FDA, one of our Nation's oldest consumer protection agencies, assures the safety of foods and cosmetics and the safety and efficacy of pharmaceuticals, biological products and medical devices. Its employees monitor the manufacture, import, transport, storage and sale of about $1 trillion worth of products each year.

Health Resources and Services Administration (HRSA)
HRSA directs national health programs that improve the Nation's health by assuring equitable access to comprehensive, quality healthcare for all. It works to improve and extend life for people living with HIV/AIDS, provide primary healthcare to medically underserved people, serve women and children through state programs, and train a health workforce that is both diverse and motivated to work in underserved communities.

Indian Health Service (IHS)
IHS is the principal Federal healthcare advocate and provider for American Indians and Alaska Natives who belong to more than 550 Federally recognized tribes in 35 states. It provides comprehensive healthcare services, including preventive, curative, rehabilitative and environmental.

National Institutes of Health (NIH)
NIH with its 27 separate components, mainly Institutes and Centers, is one of the world's foremost medical research centers, and the Federal focal

point for medical research in the U.S. Its mission is to uncover new knowledge that will lead to better health for everyone by: conducting research in its own laboratories; supporting the research of non-Federal scientists in universities, medical schools, hospitals, and research institutions throughout the Country and abroad; helping in the training of research investigators; and fostering communication of medical information.

Substance Abuse and Mental Health Services Administration (SAMHSA)
SAMHSA works to improve the quality and availability of prevention, treatment and rehabilitative services in order to reduce illness, disability, death, and cost to society resulting from substance abuse and mental illness.

Other Agencies or OpDivs of the HHS
to which PHS Officers are Assigned

Office of Public Health and Science (OPHS)
The OPHS is under the direction of the Assistant Secretary of Health, who serves as a senior advisor on public health and science issues to the Secretary of HHS. The office serves as the focal point of leadership and coordination across the Department in public health and science; provides direction to program offices with OPHS; and provides advice and counsel on public health and science issues to the Secretary.

Program Support Center (PSC)
The PSC is a service-for-fee organization that utilizes a pioneering business enterprise approach to provide government support services throughout HHS, as well as other Departments and Federal agencies.

Non-PHS Agencies and Programs
to which PHS Officers are Assigned

Bureau of Prisons (BOP)
The mission of BOP, as part of the Department of Justice, is to protect society by confining offenders in the controlled environments of prisons and community-based facilities that are safe, humane, appropriately secure, and which provide work and other self-improvement opportunities to assist offenders in becoming law-abiding citizens. PHS commissioned officers work for the Health Services Division.

Centers for Medicare and Medicaid Services (CMS)
CMS administers the Medicare and Medicaid programs which provide healthcare to America's aged and indigent populations, and the State Children's Health Insurance Program. In addition, it performs a number of quality-focused activities, including regulation of laboratory testing, development of coverage policies and quality-of-care improvement. It maintains oversight of the survey and certification of nursing homes and

continuing care providers (including home health agencies, intermediate care facilities for the mentally retarded and hospitals).

District of Columbia Commission on Mental Health Services (CMHS)
The CMHS works toward establishing a community-based system of care for the mentally ill of Washington D.C.

Environmental Protection Agency (EPA)
EPA implements the Federal laws designed to promote public health by protecting our Nation's air, water and soil from harmful pollution. EPA endeavors to accomplish its mission by systematic integration of a variety of research, monitoring, standard-setting and enforcement activities. EPA also coordinates and supports research and anti-pollution activities of state and local governments, private and public groups, individuals and educational institutions. EPA also monitors the operations of other Federal agencies with respect to their impact on the environment. PHS officers provide technical expertise in all major EPA program areas.

Federal Emergency Management Agency (FEMA)
FEMA is a component of the Department of Homeland Security. The Agency is tasked with planning for, responding to, and recovering from any national disaster. PHS officers provide technical support to FEMA.

National Oceanic and Atmospheric Administration (NOAA)
NOAA is responsible for conducting research and gathering data about the global oceans, atmosphere and space. NOAA predicts changes in the earth's environment, forecasts weather patterns and warns of dangerous weather; charts the seas and skies; and guides the use and protection of ocean and coastal resources. PHS officers provide health care services to NOAA commissioned officers and their dependents, active duty NOAA Wage Marine personnel, and certain retirees and their dependents.

National Park Service (NPS)
NPS was established to preserve the natural and cultural resources and values of the national parks for the enjoyment, education and inspiration of this and future generations. It administers more than 378 national parks, monuments, historic sites and other areas covering almost 80 million acres. PHS Commissioned Corps officers (primarily environmental health officers and engineers) provide consultative services to the NPS.

U.S. Citizenship and Immigration Services (USCIS)
USCIS, a component of the Department of Homeland Security, administers the Nation's immigration laws. It conducts immigration inspections of travelers entering (or seeking entry) the U.S. as they arrive at official ports of entry; regulates permanent and temporary immigration to the U.S.; maintains control of U.S. borders; and identifies and removes people who have no lawful immigration status. Public Health Service commissioned officers are assigned to the Division of Immigration Health Services (DIHS). DIHS provides or arranges cost-effective health service

for the delivery of direct primary healthcare detainees at Service Processing Centers or at locations throughout the Nation where detainees are being held. DIHS also provides medical consultation, technical assistance regarding detainee's healthcare, provides medical escorts for international and domestic air transport operations, and deploys medical teams on domestic and international missions.

U.S. Coast Guard (USCG)
USCG is a component of the Department of Homeland Security. The USCG is one of the seven uniformed services and is the smallest of the five armed services. Its goals are to respond to calls for help at sea; provide search and rescue; protect America's ecologically rich and sensitive marine environment; facilitate the movement of people and goods on the U.S. waterways; serve as America's principal maritime law enforcement agency; and fulfill national security missions. PHS commissioned officers provide healthcare services to USCG active duty members, dependents and retirees.

U.S. Department of Agriculture (USDA)
The USDA supports the production of agriculture by ensuring a safe, affordable, nutritious and accessible food supply; caring for agricultural, forest and range lands; supporting development of rural communities; providing economic opportunities for farm and rural residents; expanding global markets for agricultural and forest products and services; and working to reduce hunger in the U.S. and the world. PHS commissioned officers work in the Food Safety and Inspection Services program.

U.S. Marshals Service (USMS)
USMS, an agency of the Department of Justice (DOJ), protects the Federal courts and ensures the effective operation of the judicial system; investigates fugitive matters; provides for the security, health and safety of government witnesses and their immediate dependents; offers for public sale property which has been forfeited under laws enforced or administered by the DOJ; and houses and transports prisoners. PHS commissioned officers work in four USMS program areas: flight nurses aboard the Justice Prisoner and Alien Transportation system (JPATS) aircraft; coordinators of the JPATS movement of prisoners with health problems; managers of prisoner healthcare issues in the Office of Interagency Medical Services; and providers of medical support to the USMS Special Operations Group.

Policy Advisory Council

See the Surgeon General's Policy Advisory Council (SGPAC) in the Section, Special Duty.

Regular Corps

All newly appointed PHS officers are commissioned in the active Reserve Corps. Upon completing a minimum of two years of continuous active duty in their current tour (i.e., since their most recent entry into the PHS), Reserve Corps officers may request consideration for appointment and assimilation into the Regular Corps of PHS.

The Regular Corps is the career component of the PHS Commissioned Corps and is comprised of officers who have expressed long-term commitment to the missions and goals of the Corps. Because it is limited to a total of 2,800 officers as set by Congress, appointment to the Regular Corps is a selective process. The Regular Corps provides officers certain advantages in relation to the Reserve Corps. Chief among these are the following.

- Regular Corps officers have retention priority when there is a reduction-in-strength of the active duty Corps.
- Regular Corps officers are eligible for consideration for appointment as a Chief Professional Officer (Reserve officers are not eligible).
- Regular Corps officers are eligible for consideration for promotion to temporary flag rank grades (Reserve officers are not eligible).
- Regular Corps officers are eligible to be retained in the PHS beyond 30 years if justification is made by their operating division and it is approved by a PHS retention board (Reserve Corps officers are not eligible).

Reserve officers who meet the time-in-service eligibility criterion and who want to assimilate into the Regular Corps are advised to apply early in their careers. The assimilation process often requires a few years to complete due to the need for nomination by the President and confirmation by the U.S. Senate. Additionally, officers who wait until late in their careers before applying for assimilation may be passed over at the outset, because the PHS believes that an officer's intention to make a career commitment to the PHS should be set and declared early in the officer's service life.

PHS History

The origins of the United States Public Health Service (PHS) can be traced to 1798, when President John Adams signed *An Act for the Relief of Sick and Disabled Seamen,* that provided for the care and relief of sick and injured merchant seamen. The earliest marine hospitals created to care for the seamen were located along the East Coast, with Boston being the site of the first such facility; later they were also established along inland waterways, the Great Lakes and the Gulf and Pacific Coasts.

Reorganization in 1870 converted the loose network of locally controlled hospitals into a centrally controlled Marine Hospital Service, with its headquarters in Washington, D.C. The position of Supervising Surgeon (later Surgeon General) was created to administer the Service, and John Maynard Woodworth was appointed as the first incumbent in 1871. He moved quickly to reform the system and adopted a military model for his medical staff, instituting examinations for applicants and putting his physicians in uniforms. Woodworth created a cadre of mobile, career service physicians who could be assigned as needed to the various marine hospitals. The uniformed services component of the Marine Hospital Service was formalized as the Commissioned Corps when, in 1889, President Grover Cleveland signed *An Act to Regulate Appointments in the Marine Hospital Service of the United States.* The Corps was established along military lines to be a mobile force of professionals subject to reassignment to meet the needs of the Service. Originally, the Corps was composed only of physicians. However, over the course of the twentieth century, as the functional responsibilities of the Public Health Service and the Corps broadened, the Corps expanded to include dentists, sanitarians, engineers, pharmacists, nurses, sanitarians, scientists, and other health professionals.

The scope of activities of the Marine Hospital Service also began to expand well beyond the care of merchant seamen in the closing decades of the nineteenth century, beginning with the control of infectious disease. Responsibility for quarantine was originally a function of the states rather than the Federal government, but the National Quarantine Act of 1878 conferred quarantine authority on the Marine Hospital Service. Over the course of the next half a century, the Marine Hospital Service increasingly took over quarantine functions from state authorities.

As immigration increased dramatically in the late nineteenth century, the Federal government also took over the processing of immigrants from the states, beginning in 1891. The Marine Hospital Service was assigned the responsibility for the medical inspection of arriving immigrants at sites such as Ellis Island in New York. Commissioned officers played a major role in fulfilling the service's commitment to prevent disease from entering the Country.

Because of the broadening responsibilities of the Service, its name was changed in 1902 to the Public Health and Marine Hospital Service, and again in 1912 to just the Public Health Service. The Service continued to expand its public health activities as the Nation entered the twentieth century, with the Commissioned Corps leading the way. As the century progressed, PHS commissioned officers served their Country by controlling the spread of contagious diseases such as smallpox and yellow fever, conducting important biomedical research, regulating the food and drug supply, providing health care to underserved groups, supplying medical assistance in the aftermath of disasters, and in numerous other ways.

As we embark upon a new century, the PHS continues to fulfill its mission to protect and advance the public's health. It has grown from a small collection of marine hospitals to the largest public health program in the world.

PHS Flag

The PHS flag has a yellow background (gold hue) with a blue PHS seal centered on the flag. It appears to have evolved from the yellow quarantine flag used by the Service on quarantine vessels and stations. By the early twentieth century, the PHS had added its seal to the traditional yellow flag and a version of that came to be used in connection with PHS activities. By the late 1960s, specifications for the flag were formally established. The blue color represent the origins of the PHS in maritime activities.

PHS Seal

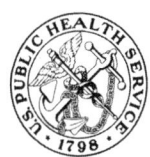

The PHS seal was originally designed by John Maynard Woodworth, who was appointed in 1871 as the first Supervising Surgeon (title was later changed to Surgeon General) of the Marine Hospital Service. The seal features a caduceus crossed with a fouled anchor, and it originally carried the words "U.S. Marine Hospital Service" with the dates 1798-1871. The 1798 date refers to the year of passage of the *Act for the Relief of Sick and Disabled Seamen,* which set up the marine hospital system that evolved into the PHS.

Today's seal is similar, except that it carries the words "U.S. Public Health Service" and only one date, 1798. The fouled anchor signifies a seaman in distress or a sick seaman. Although the caduceus is often used as a symbol of medicine, the particular symbolic form used by Woodworth is more often associated with the god Mercury to represent trade or commerce, and it is surmised that this was used due to the Service's relationship with merchant seamen and the maritime industry.

PHS CC Seal

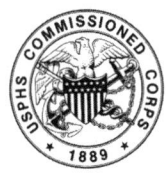

The PHS Commissioned Corps seal features the PHS service crest, and carries the words "USPHS Commissioned Corps" with the date 1889. The 1889 date refers to the year of passage of the *Act to Regulate Appointments in the Marine Hospital Service of the United States,* which formalized the Commissioned Corps.

PHS March

The "U.S. Public Health Service March" was composed by Senior Chief Musician George King III, U.S. Coast Guard. The copyright was conveyed to the Surgeon General in 1978. The words are as follows.

> The mission of our Service is known the world around.
> In research and in treatment no equal can be found.
> In the silent war against disease no truce is ever seen.
> We serve on the land and the sea for humanity,
> The Public Health Service team!

PHS Coin

The military coin is used by service personnel throughout the world as a form of recognition. The coin, also known as a *challenge* or *recognition coin,* is unique to a member's unit or uniformed service—it carries a likeness of the unit/service crest or insignia and may include its motto. The coin engenders an identity with, and camaraderie within one's own organization and among all service members who have served their Country with pride and distinction. In the PHS, officers carry the coin to "show their colors" when around colleagues and other military members. PHS coins are also used as appreciation gifts and mementos for presentation to supporters of the Corps.

There are various theories about how the coin evolved to become a symbol of military recognition. By most accounts, the tradition began during World War I when an American pilot ordered medallions struck that bore his squadron's insignia, which he presented to fellow pilots. He subsequently needed to establish his identify after escaping German capture and then being mistaken by the French as a German saboteur—his only identification was his medallion, the insignia of which was recognized by a French guard. It became a tradition for pilots to carry a recognition coin at all times. Pilots would challenge one another to produce the coin, and the tradition of a coin check came about as the way to ensure that other service members carry their coin. The challenger holds his/her coin in the air, announcing "coin check" and/or drops the coin on a table, and those challenged must show their own coin. By custom, those not having a coin are obliged to buy the challenger a drink.

The Public Health Service Coin was developed by the District of Columbia Branch, Commissioned Officers Association. The PHS Coin is approximately 1½ inches in diameter. One side has a 4-color enamel surface displaying the PHS seal and the other side displays the PHS Commissioned Corps seal. The coin is finely detailed, and the face, borders and edges are bright gold finish.

SECTION IX.
UNIFORMED SERVICE ORGANIZATIONS

There are seven uniformed services of the United States: the Public Health Service, National Oceanic and Atmospheric Administration, Air Force, Army, Coast Guard, Marine Corps, and Navy. The last five services are considered armed forces/services. All uniformed services have the common objective of providing security to the United States, and all follow similar conventions. Yet, each service has characteristics that identify it as a unique service organization. The following information is provided to highlight the organization of each service. All uniformed services have a proud record of service to the Nation, and readers are encouraged to learn more about them. The following information is derived from Department of Defense and uniformed service publications.

ORGANIZATION OF ALL MILITARY SERVICES
U.S. AIR FORCE
U.S. ARMY
U.S. COAST GUARD
U.S. MARINE CORPS
U.S. NAVY
NATIONAL OCEANIC & ATMOSPHERIC ADMINISTRATION CORPS

Organization of All Military Services

The President of the United States is the Commander in Chief of all uniformed services. With regard to national security involving the armed services, the President is advised by the Secretary of Defense, Joint Chiefs of Staff and the National Security Council. The Joint Chiefs of Staff are comprised of the top military officers—the Army Chief of Staff, the Air Force Chief of Staff, Chief of Naval Operations, and the Commandant of the Marine Corps. Presently, the military services have a combined strength of about 1.5 million active duty and 1.2 million Reserve and National Guard personnel.

The Department of Defense (DoD) was formed from the Department of War as a result of the National Security Act of 1947 (which formalized the National Military Establishment) and the National Security Act Amendments of 1949. Reporting to the DoD are three military departments, the Army, Air Force and Navy (the Marine Corps is part of the Navy), and 16 defense agencies established for specific purposes (e.g., Defense Intelligence Agency).

The armed services are operationally subordinate to their military departments, each of which is directed by a civilian Secretary appointed by the President. In addition, the departments have a senior officer who commands the respective service—the Army Chief of Staff, Air Force Chief of Staff, Chief of Naval Operations, and Commandant of the Marine Corps—who work with their department's Secretary to implement the DoD mission.

The military departments recruit, train and equip their forces. The operational control of those forces is assigned to one of nine unified commands, which are composed of two or more of the armed services:

U.S. European Command (EUCOM), Stuttgart-Vaihingen, Germany
U.S. Pacific Command (PACOM), Honolulu, Hawaii
U.S. Joint Forces Command (JFCOM), Norfolk, Virginia
U.S. Southern Command (SOUTHCOM), Miami, Florida
U.S. Central Command (CENTCOM), MacDill AFB, Florida
U.S. Northern Command (NORTHCOM), Peterson AFB, Colorado
U.S. Special Operations Command (SOCOM), MacDill AFB, Florida
U.S. Strategic Command (STRATCOM), Offutt AFB, Nebraska
U.S. Transportation Command (TRANSCOM), Scott AFB, Illinois

The Coast Guard resides organizationally within the Department of Homeland Security and is commanded by the Coast Guard Commandant. The National Oceanic and Atmospheric Administration (NOAA) is in the Department of Commerce and is commanded by the Director, NOAA Commissioned Corps. In times of national emergency, including war, the President can transfer any or all Coast Guard assets to the Department of the Navy, and PHS and NOAA assets to any of the armed services.

U.S. Air Force

Organization
The Department of the Air Force is responsible for conducting military operations in air and space. It is administered by a civilian Secretary appointed by the President, and it is supervised by a military Chief of Staff appointed by the President with the consent of the Senate for a four-year term. The Secretary and Chief of Staff together direct the Air Force mission.

The Secretary of the Air Force is responsible for the conduct of all affairs of the Air Force, including administration, training, operations, logistical support and maintenance, personnel welfare, and research and development. The Chief of Staff of the Air Force presides over the Air Staff, transmits plans and recommendations to the Secretary and acts as the Secretary's agent in carrying them out. The Chief of Staff is responsible for the preparedness of its forces for military operations and supervises the administration of Air Force personnel assignments. The Chief of Staff also serves as a member of the Joint Chiefs of Staff and the Armed Forces Policy Council.

Current personnel strength of the Air Force is about 350,000 active duty members, plus two Reserve components—the Air Force Reserve and the Air National Guard with a combined strength of about 200,000 personnel. There are nine major commands, organized on a functional basis within the U.S. and by geographic location elsewhere. There are 35 field operating agencies and four direct reporting units. The basic organizational unit is a squadron, with between 8 and 24 aircraft depending on whether it is a bomber, fighter, or transport squadron; four or more squadrons form a wing, which is the basic combat unit; two or more wings form an air division; and, two or more divisions comprise a numbered air force.

Virtually the entire Air Force is further divided into ten Aerospace Expeditionary Forces (AEFs), with each force composed of about the same air and space capability and approximately 10,000 to 15,000 personnel. Each AEF maintains readiness for immediate deployment for 120 days every 20 months, and two of the ten AEFs are on call at any one time. This approach allows the Air Force to better manage its resources in responding to worldwide contingencies.

Mission
The mission of the Air Force is to defend the United States and protect its interests through aerospace power.

Organizational History
The Air Force is the youngest of the armed forces, having been formally established in 1947. Its origins began in 1907 as the Aeronautical Division of the U.S. Army Signal Corps. The progress of American aviation was slow, however, with Congress voting an appropriation for the first time in 1911 and

authorizing creation of the Army Aviation Section of the Signal Corps in 1914. The name changed to the Air Service in 1918 and then to the Army Air Corps in 1926, which became a subordinate element of the Army Air Forces in 1941 and continued as a combat arm of the Army until 1947. In 1947, President Truman signed the National Security Act which provided for a new defense organization, DoD, and a separate Department of the Air Force. The important role of military aviation was proven during its use in World Wars I and II. The Air Force's combat role advanced from tactical support of ground forces to include strategic bombing and maintenance of U.S. nuclear forces.

U.S. Army

Organization
The Department of the Army is responsible for conducting military operations on land. It is administered by a civilian Secretary appointed by the President, and it is supervised by a military Chief of Staff appointed by the President with the consent of the Senate for a four year term. The Secretary and Chief of Staff together direct the Army mission. The Secretary of the Army and Chief of Staff have responsibilities very similar to those of their counterparts in the Air Force. The Chief of Staff also serves as a member of the Joint Chiefs of Staff and the Armed Forces Policy Council.

The U.S. Army is comprised of the Regular Army, with about 500,000 active duty personnel, and two Reserve components—the Federal Army Reserve with about 200,000 personnel; and, the individual state-based Army National Guard with about 350,000 personnel. The President or Secretary of Defense can activate state National Guard units into Federal military service when needed. There are nine major field commands that carry out the mission of the Army.

The Army's combat units are called divisions. Currently, there are about ten active (armored, mechanized, infantry, airborne, air assault) and eight Reserve divisions, each consisting of about 11,000 to 16,000 soldiers. Each division includes support units, such as communications and supply, so that it is able to operate independently. A division contains three or more brigades or regiments with 3,000 to 5,000 soldiers; each brigade has three to five battalions of 500 to 1,200 soldiers; each battalion has three or more companies, batteries (field artillery) or troops (cavalry) with about 150 soldiers, which are organized into platoons of approximately 40 soldiers.

Mission
The mission of the Army is to fight and win our Nation's wars by providing prompt, sustained land dominance across the full range of military operations and spectrum of conflict in support of combatant commanders.

Organizational History

The Army is the oldest U.S. military service, with origins in the Continental Army which was established on June 14, 1775 at the outset of the Revolutionary War. Members of the Army were split during the American Civil War (1861–1865) between Union and Confederate forces. National Guard units trace their lineage to the 1600s when three colonial militia units were formed in Massachusetts.

U.S. Coast Guard

Organization

The Coast Guard (CG) is a branch of the armed forces that is responsible for protecting the Nation's interests in its ports and waterways, along its coastlines and in international waters. Its responsibilities can be broadly categorized as ensuring maritime safety, enforcing maritime security, protecting natural resources, and national defense. The Coast Guard resides organizationally within the Department of Homeland Security. A Coast Guard Commandant at headquarters in Washington, D.C. oversees all operations and supervises two major command areas: the CG Pacific Area, headquartered in Alameda, California, and the CG Atlantic Area, headquartered in Portsmouth, Virginia. The two command areas are divided into nine geographic districts for specific regions of the Nation.

Current personnel strength is about 39,000 active duty personnel and 8,000 members in the CG Reserve.

Approximately 32,000 civilian volunteers comprise the Coast Guard Auxiliary. The Auxiliary was authorized by act of Congress in 1939, and is comprised of civilian volunteers who assist the CG in performing any function, duty, role, mission or operation. They are probably best known for educating the public through boating safety classes.

During war times and upon direction of the President, the Coast Guard serves as part of the Navy.

Mission

The mission of the Coast Guard is to protect the public, the environment, and U.S. economic interests—in the Nation's ports and waterways, along the coast, on international waters, or in any maritime region as required to support national security.

Organizational History

The Coast Guard traces its history back to August 4, 1790 when the first Congress authorized the construction of ten vessels to enforce tariff and trade laws, prevent smuggling, and protect the collection of the Federal revenue. Known variously as the Revenue Marine and the Revenue Cutter Service, the

Coast Guard greatly expanded in size and responsibilities, to include humanitarian duties and law enforcement functions, as the Nation grew.

The Coast Guard was formed in 1915 under an act of Congress when the Revenue Cutter Service was merged with the Life-Saving Service. The new organization operated under the direction of the Department of the Treasury during peace time, and as part of the Navy in wartime.

The Lighthouse Service was transferred to the Coast Guard in 1939. Later, in 1946, Congress transferred the Bureau of Marine Inspection and Navigation to the Coast Guard, thereby placing merchant marine licensing and merchant vessel safety under its purview. In 1967, the CG was transferred to the Department of Transportation until 2002, when Congress approved legislation transferring it to the Department of Homeland Security.

U.S. Marine Corps

Organization

The Marine Corps is responsible for rapid troop deployment for combined land, sea, and air operations. The Marine Corps also provides security on Navy ships and bases, and at U.S. embassies abroad. The Corps is a separate service within the Department of the Navy. Administered by a civilian Secretary of the Navy, the Corps is supervised by a military Commandant of the Marine Corps who is a member of the Joint Chiefs of Staff.

The principal operating forces of the Marine Corps are the fleet Marine Forces and security forces. The Corps is combat-organized into Marine air-ground task forces (MAGTFs). The largest MAGTFs are three Marine Expeditionary Forces (MEFs), each of which has rapid deployment combat forces called Marine Expeditionary Units. The MEFs are stationed at Camp Lejeune, North Carolina; Camp Pendleton, California; and in Okinawa, Japan. Current personnel strength of the Marine Corps is about 175,000 active duty and 40,000 Marine Corps Reserve members.

Organizational History

The Marine Corps traces its beginning to November 10, 1775, when the Continental Congress passed a resolution stating that "two Battalions of Marines be raised" for service as landing forces with the naval fleet. The Revolutionary War ended in 1783, and the Marines were reactivated in 1798 by an act of Congress. The National Security Act of 1947 reaffirmed the Corps' status as an independent service.

U.S. Navy

Organization
The Department of the Navy is the maritime military force, responsible for deploying personnel on board ships, submarines and aircraft to strike on the sea or land. It is administered by a civilian secretary appointed by the President and supervised by a military Chief of Naval Operations appointed by the President with the consent of the Senate for a four year term. The Secretary and Chief together direct the Navy mission, and have responsibilities very similar to those of their counterparts in the Air Force. The Chief also serves as a member of the Joint Chiefs of Staff and the Armed Forces Policy Council.

Since World War II, the Navy has maintained fleets in the Atlantic Ocean and Mediterranean Sea, designated with even numbers, and in the Pacific Ocean, with odd numbers. A few of these fleets are assigned to unified commands, with the others remaining under the jurisdiction of the Department of the Navy. There is presently a major base at Jacksonville, Florida, and five operating forces:

    The Second Fleet (Atlantic), Norfolk, Virginia
    The Third Fleet (Eastern/Northern Pacific), San Diego, California
    The Fifth Fleet (Persian Gulf, Middle East), Manama, Bahrain
    The Sixth Fleet (Mediterranean), Gaeta, Italy
    The Seventh Fleet (Western Pacific, Indian Ocean), Yokusuka, Japan

Current personnel strength of the Navy is about 375,000 active duty and 450,000 Naval Reserve members.

Mission
The mission of the Navy is to be organized, trained and equipped primarily for prompt and sustainable combat incident to operations at sea.
Navy Regulations, art. 0202.

Organizational History
The Navy's origins began when, on October 13, 1775, the Continental Congress voted to fit out two sailing vessels for the purpose of intercepting transports carrying supplies to the British Army. The Constitution of the U.S., ratified in 1789, empowers Congress to "provide and maintain a Navy." From 1794 until 1798, administration of naval affairs was the responsibility of the Department of War. In 1798, Congress established the Department of the Navy. The National Security Act of 1947 created the Department of Defense, to include the military Departments.

National Oceanic and Atmospheric Administration Corps

Organization
The National Oceanic and Atmospheric Administration (NOAA) is administered by the U.S. Department of Commerce. The NOAA Commissioned Corps is directed by a senior commissioned officer who also serves as Deputy Director of NOAA Marine and Aviation Operations. The role of commissioned officers is to operate NOAA's fleet of research and survey vessels and aircraft, and serve in administrative and scientific posts within NOAA.

Current personnel strength of the NOAA Corps is about 300 active duty commissioned officers.

Mission
The mission of the NOAA Corps is to provide officers technically competent to assume positions of leadership and command in the NOAA and Department of Commerce programs, and in the armed forces during times of war or national emergency.

Organizational History
The NOAA Corps is the "seventh" uniformed service. NOAA traces its lineage to 1807 when President Thomas Jefferson signed a bill for the "Survey of the Coast." This resulted in formation of the U.S. Coast and Geodetic Survey (C&GS, or Coast Survey), the oldest scientific agency in the Federal government. Before the Civil War, the work force of the Coast Survey was made up of civilians, along with Army and Naval officers. With the outbreak of the Civil War, most all military officers were withdrawn and the civilian surveyors, by virtue of their service on the war's front lines, were the predecessors of today's NOAA Corps. With the entry of the U.S. into the First World War, the commissioned service of the C&GS was formed, thereby assuring the rapid assimilation of technical skills for defense purposes. Following two reorganizations in which various science agencies were brought together, the NOAA and NOAA Corps came into existence in 1970.

Abbreviations, Acronyms & Glossary

Air Mobility Command (AMC) – The Air Force component of the U.S. Transportation Command.
ASG – Assistant Surgeon General
As you were – The order to resume the previous activity.
Attaché – An expert representative on the diplomatic staff of his/her country at a foreign capitol.
Attention on deck – The call given by the officer who sees a senior officer entering the room.
Aye, aye – The response to an order indicating that the order was heard, understood, and will be carried out.
BDU – Battle dress uniform
BOQ – Bachelor officer quarters
BOTC – Basic Officer Training Course
BPED – Base pay entry date
Bravo Zulu – The phonetic pronunciation of BZ, from the NATO signal codes, meaning "Well done."
BX – Base exchange
CAD – Call to active duty (date)
Carry on – The order to resume the previous activity.
CCPM – Commissioned Corps Personnel Manual
CCRF – Commissioned Corps Readiness Force
Chargé d' Affaires – The officer in charge of diplomatic business in the absence of the ambassador or minister.
CO – Commanding officer
Colors – The national flag; the distinguishing flag flown to indicate a ship's nationality; the Naval ceremonies of hoisting the national flag at 0800 and hauling it down at sunset.
Commission – Written order granting an officer rank and authority; to activate a ship or station.
Company grade – Refers to officers of the 0-1 to 0-3 grades in the Air Force, Army, and Marine Corps.
CONUS – Continental United States
COTA – Commissioned Officer Training Academy
CPO – Chief Professional Officer
DBDU – Desert battle dress uniform

DHHS – Department of Health and Human Services
DOD – Department of Defense
DSG – Deputy Surgeon General
DV – Distinguished visitor
Ensign – The national flag; the flag flown to indicate a military ship's nationality; the most junior commissioned officer rank in the Navy, Coast Guard, NOAA, and USPHS.
EOD – Entry on duty
Field grade – Refers to officers of the 0-4 to 0-6 grades in the Air Force, Army, and Marine Corps.
Flag officer – Admiral or General (pay grade 0-7 and above) in the uniformed services.
General officer – General (pay grade 0-7 and above) in the Air Force, Army, and Marine Corps.
Hail and farewell – A social function to welcome newcomers and bid farewell to those leaving a duty station.
HQ – Headquarters
Interoperability – The term used to indicate the capability of uniformed services to act in conjunction with one another to complete a mission.
IOTC – Independent Officer Training Course
JOAG – Junior Officer Advisory Group
Junior officer – Refers to officers of the 0-1 to 0-4 grades in the Coast Guard, Navy, NOAA, and PHS.
Line officer – Refers to an officer who is trained to assume command in a combat situation.
LUA – Local Uniform Authority
MAC – Military Airlift Command
Merchant ensign – The flag flown to indicate a merchant ship's nationality.
Mess – The area or room where meals are served.
MOLC – Minority Officers Liaison Council
Morning and evening colors – Naval term for the daily ceremony of raising and lowering the national flag.
MPF – Military personnel flight
MRE – Meal, ready-to-eat
NASA – National Aeronautics and Space Administration
NATO – North Atlantic Treaty Organization
NCO – Noncommissioned officer
OASH – Office of the Assistant Secretary for Health, HHS
OCCFM – Office of Commissioned Corps Force Management
OCCO – Office of Commissioned Corps Operations

OCONUS – Outside the continental United States
OFRD – Office of Force Readiness and Deployment
OIC – Officer in charge
OOD – Officer of the deck; a senior petty officer, warrant or commissioned officer who stands at the entry point to a ship, and who grants permission to come aboard or depart the ship.
OpDiv – Operating division/agency/program
OPF – Official personnel folder
OPHS – Office of Public Health and Science
ORA – Office of Reserve Affairs
OSC – Office of Science and Communications
OSG – Office of the Surgeon General
PAC – Professional Advisory Committee
PAO – Public affairs officer
Pay grade – Alphanumeric designation that corresponds to the seniority of a service member. *O* designates a commissioned officer, *W* a warrant officer, and *E* an enlisted member.
PCS – Permanent change of (duty) station
PX – Post exchange (Army)
Quarterdeck – The area of a ship where the OOD stands watch; this is normally on the main deck near the gangway.
Rate – Naval term for an enlisted member's rank or pay grade.
Rating – Naval term for an enlisted member's occupational specialty.
Regular Corps – The career component of the PHS Commissioned Corps. Reserve Corps officers must request appointment into the Regular Corps.
Reserve Corps – The active reserve component of the PHS Commissioned Corps. Newly appointed officers are commissioned in the Reserve Corps.
Reveille and retreat – Army and Air Force term for the daily ceremony of raising and lowering the national flag.
ROG – Research Officers Group
Senior officer – Refers to officers at the 0-5 to 0-6 grades in the Coast Guard, Navy, NOAA, and PHS.
SG – Surgeon General
SGPAC – Surgeon General's Policy Advisory Council
Smoking lamp – During the days of sailing ships, a lamp from which to light cigars or pipes. In current usage, the phrase *The smoking lamp is lighted* means that smoking is permitted.
TAD – Temporary additional duty
TDY – Temporary duty
TRANSCOM – U.S. Transportation Command

Very well – The reply of a senior officer to a junior officer's verbal report; never said by a junior to a senior officer.
VOQ – Visiting officer quarters
XO – Executive officer, who is second in command.
Zulu time – Greenwich Mean Time (GMT).

SELECTED REFERENCES

NOTE: Approximately 100 sources of protocol, etiquette, and service standards information and regulations were used in the preparation of the *Public Health Service Officer's Guide*. The references which follow are among the most reliable sources of information.

Publications

Air Education and Training Command. *Protocol Primer.* Pamphlet 90-101. Headquarters. Washington, DC. 1 November 1995.

Air Force Space Command. *'Til Wheels are Up.* Protocol Office. Luke Air Force Base. Unofficial protocol document of the US Air Force.

Baldrige L. *New Complete Guide to Executive Manners.* New York: Rawson Associates. 1993.

Baldrige L. *New Manners for New Times.* New York: Scribner. 2003.

Benton JC. *Air Force Officer's Guide.* 33rd Ed. Mechanicsburg, PA: Stackpole Books. 2002.

Bonn, KE. *Army Officer's Guide.* 49th Ed. Mechanicsburg, PA: Stackpole Books. 2002.

Connell RW, Mack WP. *Naval Ceremonies, Customs, and Traditions.* 6th Ed. Annapolis: Naval Institute Press. 2004.

Department of the Air Force. *Handbook for Generals' Aides.* Air Force Manual 36-6. Headquarters. Washington, DC.

Department of the Army. *A Guide to Protocol and Etiquette for Official Entertainment.* Pamphlet 600-60. Headquarters. Washington, DC. 11 December 2001.

Department of the Army. *Drill and Ceremonies.* Field Manual No. 3-21.5. Headquarters. Washington, DC. 7 July 2003.

Department of the Army. *Army Leadership.* Field Manual No. 22-100. Headquarters. Washington, DC. 31 August 1999.

Department of the Army. *Preparing and Managing Correspondence.* Army Regulation 25-50. Headquarters. Washington, DC. 3 June 2002.

Department of the Army. *Salutes, Honors, and Visits of Courtesy.* Army Regulation 600-25. Headquarters. Washington, DC. 1 September 1983.

Department of the Navy. *Social Usage and Protocol Handbook. A Guide for Personnel of the U.S. Navy.* OPNAVINST 1710.7A. Office of the Chief of Naval Operations. Washington, DC. 15 June 2001.

Department of the Navy. Naval School. Civil Engineer Corps Officers. *Mess Night Manual.* Port Hueneme, CA. August 1986.

Ford C. *21st Century Etiquette.* New York: The Lyons Press. 2001.

Knoben JE, Knoben LH. *Executive Etiquette: Contemporary Etiquette and Business Practice for the Professional Person.* Hamilton, IL: DI Publications/Hamilton Press. 1990.

Mack WP, Seymour Jr HA, McComas LA. *The Naval Officer's Guide. 11th Ed.* Annapolis: Naval Institute Press. 1998.

Moore JH. *The Etiquette Advantage.* Nashville: Broadman & Holman Publishers. 1998.

Mullan F. *Plagues and Politics.* New York: Basic Books Publishers. 1989.

Naval Computer and Telecommunications Station. *Transferring to the Fleet Reserve/Retirement.* Washington, DC. 1999.

Office of Personnel Management. *Guide to Senior Executive Service Qualifications.* Washington, DC. 1998.

Post P. *Emily Post's Etiquette. 17th Ed.* New York: Harper Resource. 2004.

Post P, Post P. *The Etiquette Advantage in Business. 2nd Ed.* New York: Harper Resource. 2005.

Robert HM, Evans WJ, Honemann DH, Balch TJ. *Robert's Rules of Order. 10th Ed.* New York: Harper Collins Publishers. 2000.

Swartz OD. *Service Etiquette. 4th Ed.* Annapolis: Naval Institute Press. 1988.

US Military Academy. *Guide to Military Dining-in.* Protocol Office. West Point, NY.

US Public Health Service. *Commissioned Corps Personnel Manual.* Rockville, MD.

US Public Health Service. *Commissioned Officer's Handbook.* Rockville, MD. 1998.

Washington G. *Rules of Civility & Decent Behaviour (circa 1746).* Bedford, MA: Applewood Books. 1988.

Internet Sites

Department of Defense, Defense Link
  www.defenselink.mil
National Oceanic & Atmospheric Administration Corps
  www.noaacorps.noaa.gov
US Air Force
  www.af.mil
US Army
  www.army.mil
US Coast Guard
  www.uscg.mil
US Marine Corps
  www.usmc.mil
US Navy
  www.navy.mil
US Public Health Service
  dcp.psc.gov
  www.usphs.gov

APPENDICES

APPENDIX A.   Planning a Dining-Out
Administrative Information
Ceremony Components
Ceremony Personnel
Facility Arrangements
Meal and Reception Arrangements

APPENDIX B.   Planning a Formal Reception
Administrative Information
Reception Components
Reception Personnel
Facility Arrangements
Reception Arrangements

APPENDIX C.   Planning for
Awards/Promotion/Retirement Ceremony
Administrative Information
Type of Ceremony
Ceremony Components
Ceremony Personnel
Facility Arrangements
Reception Arrangements

APPENDIX D.   Escort Officer
Planning for a Distinguished Visitor
Administrative Information
Transportation
Accommodations
Pre-Arrival Preparations
Facility Arrangements
Event Personnel
Reception Arrangements

APPENDIX E.   Deployment
Suggested Items to Take

APPENDIX A

Planning a Dining-Out

EVENT NAME: _____
DATE, TIME: _____
PLACE: _____
SPONSOR: _____
PROGRAM COORDINATOR: _____
PRESIDING OFFICER: _____
MISTER/MADAME VICE: _____
HONORED GUEST: _____

A. CEREMONY COMPONENTS

    __√__ **ITEM COMPLETE & NOTES**
    _____ CHIMES _____
    _____ GAVEL _____
    _____ GIFTS _____
    _____ GROG BOWL _____
    _____ INVITATIONS _____
    _____ INVOCATION _____
    _____ MENU
            MENU SELECTIONS _____
            MENU PRINTED _____
    _____ PROGRAM
            PROGRAM PREPARED _____
            PROGRAM PRINTED _____
    _____ PUBLICITY _____
    _____ SCRIPT _____
    _____ TOASTS, PREARRANGED _____

APPENDIX A

B. CEREMONY PERSONNEL

    √   **ITEM COMPLETE & NOTES**

       _____ PLANNING COMMITTEE
- MEMBERS ASSIGNED _____
- DUTIES ASSIGNED _____

       _____ BAGPIPER _____
       _____ COLOR GUARD _____
       _____ MUSIC ENSEMBLE _____
       _____ PHOTOGRAPHER _____
       _____ TREASURER _____

C. FACILITY ARRANGEMENTS

    √   **ITEM COMPLETE & NOTES**

       _____ FACILITY CONTACT _____
       _____ PRE-DINNER RECEPTION ROOM _____
       _____ DINING ROOM _____
       _____ FLAGS/STANDS _____
       _____ MICROPHONES _____
       _____ MUSIC [TAPED] _____
       _____ PARKING _____
       _____ PODIUM _____
       _____ ROOM DIAGRAM _____
       _____ TABLES AND SEATING
- GENERAL _____
- HEAD TABLE _____
- VICE TABLE _____

D. MEAL AND RECEPTION ARRANGEMENTS

    √   **ITEM COMPLETE & NOTES**

       _____ BEVERAGES [ALCOHOL/NONALCOHOL] _____
       _____ CENTERPIECES _____
       _____ PLACE CARDS [HEAD TABLE] _____
       _____ PLACE SETTINGS [FORMAL] _____
       _____ TABLES/SEATING _____

APPENDIX B
PAGE 1 OF 2

Planning a Formal Reception

EVENT NAME: _____
DATE, TIME: _____
PLACE: _____
SPONSOR: _____
PROGRAM COORDINATOR: _____
HOST OFFICER: _____
HONORED GUEST: _____
HONORED GUEST SPOUSE: _____

A. RECEPTION COMPONENTS

  √ **ITEM COMPLETE & NOTES**
  ____ INVITATIONS _____
  ____ PROGRAM
     PROGRAM PREPARED _____
     PROGRAM PRINTED _____
  ____ PUBLICITY _____
  ____ RECEIVING LINE
     LOCATION IN ROOM _____
     ORDER OF PRECEDENCE _____
     ANNOUNCER _____
     END LINE OFFICER _____
     TABLE AND FLAGS _____

APPENDIX B
PAGE 2 OF 2

B. RECEPTION PERSONNEL

    √ **ITEM COMPLETE & NOTES**

    ____ PLANNING COMMITTEE
        MEMBERS ASSIGNED _____
        DUTIES ASSIGNED _____

    ____ AIDE _____

    ____ ESCORTS _____

    ____ COLOR GUARD _____

    ____ MUSIC ENSEMBLE _____

    ____ PHOTOGRAPHER _____

C. FACILITY ARRANGEMENTS

    √ **ITEM COMPLETE & NOTES**

    ____ FACILITY CONTACT _____

    ____ FLAGS / STANDS _____

    ____ MICROPHONES _____

    ____ MUSIC [TAPED] _____

    ____ PARKING _____

    ____ PODIUM _____

    ____ ROOM DIAGRAM _____

    ____ TABLE [HEAD] _____

D. RECEPTION ARRANGEMENTS

    √ **ITEM COMPLETE & NOTES**

    ____ BEVERAGES [ALCOHOL / NONALCOHOL] _____

    ____ DECORATIONS _____

    ____ MENU _____

    ____ PLACE CARDS [HEAD TABLE] _____

    ____ TABLES / SEATING _____

APPENDIX C
PAGE 1 OF 2

Planning for Awards/Promotion/Retirement Ceremony

EVENT NAME: _____
DATE, TIME: _____
PLACE: _____
SPONSOR: _____
PROGRAM COORDINATOR: _____
PRESIDING OFFICER: _____
HONORED GUEST: _____
HONORED GUEST SPOUSE: _____

A. CEREMONY COMPONENTS

    __√__ **TYPE OF CEREMONY**
    _____ DECORATION CEREMONY
            AWARDS, CITATIONS _____
    _____ PROMOTION CEREMONY
            PROMOTION ORDERS _____
            RANK INSIGNIA _____
    _____ RETIREMENT CEREMONY
            AWARD RECOGNITION _____
            RETIREE BIOGRAPHY _____
            RETIREMENT ORDERS _____
            RETIREMENT GIFTS/PRESENTATIONS _____

    __√__ **ITEM COMPLETE & NOTES**
    _____ BRIEFING FOLDER _____
    _____ INVITATIONS _____
    _____ PROGRAM
            PROGRAM PREPARED _____
            PROGRAM PRINTED _____
    _____ PUBLICITY _____
    _____ SCRIPT _____

APPENDIX C
PAGE 2 OF 2

B. CEREMONY PERSONNEL

    __√__ **ITEM COMPLETE & NOTES**
    ____ PLANNING COMMITTEE
        MEMBERS ASSIGNED _____
        DUTIES ASSIGNED _____
    ____ ADJUTANT _____
    ____ AIDE _____
    ____ COLOR GUARD _____
    ____ MUSIC ENSEMBLE _____
    ____ PHOTOGRAPHER _____
    ____ USHERS _____

C. FACILITY ARRANGEMENTS

    __√__ **ITEM COMPLETE & NOTES**
    ____ FACILITY CONTACT _____
    ____ FLAGS/STANDS _____
    ____ MICROPHONES _____
    ____ MUSIC [TAPED] _____
    ____ PARKING _____
    ____ PODIUM _____
    ____ ROOM DIAGRAM _____
    ____ STAGE SEATING _____
    ____ STAGE TABLE _____

D. RECEPTION ARRANGEMENTS

    __√__ **ITEM COMPLETE & NOTES**
    ____ BEVERAGES [ALCOHOL/NONALCOHOL] _____
    ____ CENTERPIECES _____
    ____ FOOD, SPECIAL ORDER [CAKE] _____
    ____ MENU _____
    ____ PLACE CARDS [HEAD TABLE] _____
    ____ RECEIVING LINE _____
    ____ TABLES/SEATING _____

APPENDIX D
PAGE 1 OF 3

Escort Officer
Planning for a Distinguished Visitor

DV Rank, Full Name: _____

Duty Title: _____

Duty Station: _____

Mailing Address: _____

DV Contact Numbers: _____

Dates of Visit: _____

Purpose of Visit: _____

Official Party Members (Include spouse if traveling with DV)

Rank	Full Name	Duty Title, Duty Station

Aide: _____

Escort Officer: _____

Program Coordinator: _____

A. TRANSPORTATION

    __√__ **Item Complete & Notes**

    _____ Airline Reservation Confirmation Number _____

    _____ Vehicle Reservation Confirmation Number _____

Flight Data

	Airport	Date	Time	Airline	Flight #
Arrival					
Departure					

Vehicle Data

GSA/Rental Co. Name:
GSA/Rental Co. Address:
GSA/Rental Co. Telephone Number:
Car Mfr./License Number:

APPENDIX D
PAGE 2 OF 3

B. ACCOMMODATIONS

_____ BASE/HOTEL RESERVATION CONFIRMATION NUMBER _____

LODGING DATA

BASE QUARTERS/HOTEL NAME:
BASE/HOTEL ADDRESS:
BASE/HOTEL TELEPHONE NUMBER:
CHECK-IN TIME:
CHECK-OUT TIME:

C. PRE-ARRIVAL PREPARATIONS

__√__ **ITEM COMPLETE & NOTES**

_____ GROUND TRANSPORTATION

    DRIVER ASSIGNED _____

    DRIVER BRIEFED _____

    DRIVER KNOWS DIRECTIONS _____

_____ SENIOR OFFICER AT ARRIVAL _____

_____ ITINERARY (Attach)

    COMPLETE _____

    REHEARSAL _____

_____ BRIEF FOR DV (Itinerary, Contact Information, Names, Notes)

D. FACILITY ARRANGEMENTS

__√__ **ITEM COMPLETE & NOTES**

_____ FACILITY CONTACT _____

_____ FLAGS/STANDS _____

_____ MICROPHONES _____

_____ MUSIC [TAPED] _____

_____ PARKING _____

_____ PODIUM _____

_____ ROOM DIAGRAM _____

_____ SEATING ASSIGNMENTS _____

_____ TABLE [HEAD] _____

APPENDIX D
PAGE 3 OF 3

E. **EVENT PERSONNEL**

    √ **ITEM COMPLETE & NOTES**

    ____ PLANNING COMMITTEE

        MEMBERS ASSIGNED _____

        DUTIES ASSIGNED _____

    ____ DV GREETER _____

    ____ COLOR GUARD _____

    ____ MUSIC ENSEMBLE _____

    ____ PHOTOGRAPHER _____

F. **RECEPTION ARRANGEMENTS**

    √ **ITEM COMPLETE & NOTES**

    ____ BEVERAGES [ALCOHOL/NONALCOHOL] _____

    ____ MENU _____

    ____ PLACE CARDS [HEAD TABLE] _____

    ____ RECEIVING LINE _____

    ____ TABLES/SEATING _____

APPENDIX E

Deployment Suggested Items to Take

The chart which follows is modified from an OFRD list of suggested items to take on a deployment. Officers should individualize it to meet their needs in relation to the specific deployment.

KEY
- **ALL** — This item is recommended or required for all types of deployments.
- **NORM** — Normal deployments (non-field, non-military).
- **FIELD** — Deployments to the field or in austere conditions.
- **MIL** — Deployments with a military unit.
- **OUS** — Deployments outside of the continental United States.

CATEGORY / ITEM	ALL	NORM	FIELD	MIL	OUS
Administrative					
Orders	•				
Drivers licenses (personal, military)	•				
Dog tags	•				
ID Card, USPHS	•				
ID Card, NDMS (if applicable)	•				
Notebook/pen/pencil	•				
Passport (official)					•
Food, Medical					
Food rations (one day supply)	•				
Antacids, Antihistamines	•				
Aspirin/Tylenol	•				
First aid kit (personal)	•				
Imodium (antidiarrheal)	•				
Insect repellent (pump type)			•		•
Prescription drugs (2 weeks supply)	•				
Prescription glasses (2 pairs)	•				
Sunscreen (per season)	•				
Money					
Credit card(s)	•				
Money/Travelers checks	•				
Numerous quarters	•				
Phone card	•				

Continued on next page.

APPENDIX E
PAGE 2 OF 3

Category/Item	\	DEPLOYMENT TYPE			
	ALL	NORM	FIELD	MIL	OUS
Clothing, Uniforms					
BDUs			•	•	
Boots (black combat), inserts			•	•	
Civilian/Professional		•			•
Exercise clothes, shoes	•				
Khakis, Working		•			•
Poncho/Rain jacket (light)	•				
Shoelaces (extra)	•				
Shoe shine kit	•				
Swim Suit	•				
Equipment & Field Gear					
Batteries (extra new)			•		
Bed sheet			•		
Blanket (OD, green)			•		
Canteen w/ cup (filled)			•		
Clothes line/small rope			•		
Clothes pins			•		
Compass			•		
Cup (collapsible, pocket size)			•		
Duffel bag (w/ liner, lock)			•	•	
Flashlight (black or green)			•		
Laundry bag			•		
Mosquito netting			•		
Multi-use knife (not in carry-on bag)	•				
Radio, small portable			•		
Sleeping bag			•		
Sunglasses (military type)	•				
Towels (large, small, OD/green)			•		
Watch (black waterproof)	•				
Zip Loc bags	•				

Continued on next page.

APPENDIX E

PAGE 3 OF 3

Category/Item	Deployment Type				
	All	Norm	Field	Mil	OUS
Toiletries					
Alcohol pads/Baby wipes	●				
Comb/Hair brush	●				
Deodorant (unscented)	●				
Foot powder	●				
Hand cream	●				
Handkerchiefs	●				
Lip balm (per season)	●				
Mirror (unbreakable)	●				
Sewing kit	●				
Scissors (small)	●				
Shampoo (unscented)	●				
Shaving kit	●				
Shower shoes/Flip flops	●				
Soap (in plastic container)	●				
Tissues (small packs)	●				
Toilet paper	●				
Toothbrush/paste	●				

The following items are prohibited: alcoholic beverages, earrings, electrical appliances, firearms, illegal drugs, jewelry, large sums of money, picnic coolers, purses (with BDUs), Rambo knives, sterno heaters, and tents.

NOTES

INDEX

Abbreviations and acronyms, 151
Address, forms of
    civilian, 102
    military, 29, 130
Aide-de-camp, 64
Air Force, *See* U.S. Air Force
Army, *See* U.S. Army
Attention
    coming to, 32
Awards
    order of precedence, 20
    presentation of, 53
Awards and badges, 20, 24
Bags, carrying, 16
Badges, 20, 24
Basics, uniformed service, 1
Boards, Commissioned Corps, 67
Business cards, 89
Calls, military
    official, 91
    social, 92
Cards
    attaché, 92
    business, 89
    calling, 92
    menu, 119
    personal, 92
    place, 119
Cellular phone, 106

Ceremony
    awards, 53
    dining-in, dining-out, 42
    dinners, official, 46
    promotion, 56
    protocol, 42
    receptions, 46
    retirement, 59
Chief professional officer, 68
Coast Guard, *See* U.S. Coast Guard
Coin, PHS, 142
Commissioned officer, *See* Officer
Communications
    business cards, 89
    calls and cards, 91
    conversation, 93
    correspondence, 95
    devices, carrying, 16
    greetings & introductions, 100
    invitations, 47
    presentations & speaking, 103
    telecommunications, 105
Conversation, 93
Correspondence, 95
Courtesy and protocol, *See* Military
    courtesy and protocol
Deployment
    preparation, 86
    readiness, 84

suggested items to take, 167
Device standards, 15
Dining-in, 42
Dining-out, 42
Dinners
    guest of honor, 50, 51
    host, 50, 51
    invitations, 47
    official, 46
    order of precedence, 49
    restaurant, 124
    seating arrangements, 51
    table manners, 120
    table settings, 115
    toasts, 52
Distinguished visitor, 70
Electronic mail, 105
Enlisted personnel
    qualifications, 8
    grades, insignia, ratings, 8-10
    titles, 29, 30
Escort officer, 69
Flag etiquette, 33
Foreign stations, 92
Funeral, military, 36
Glossary, 151
Greetings
    and address, 29
    and introductions, 100
Guest of honor
    dining-out, 46
    receiving line, 50
    seating arrangement, 51

Handshake, 32
Headgear
    protocol, 35
    types, 16
Honor Corps, 73
Honor position, 38
Host
    duties of, 124, 127
    receiving line, 50
    seating arrangement, 51
Insignia
    commissioned officer,
        7, 8, 12-14, 19
    enlisted, 8-10
    warrant officer, 8, 11
Introductions, 101
Invitations, 47
Junior Officer Advisory Group, 76
Leadership
    theories, 4
    attributes, skills,
        core competencies, 5
    principles and qualities, 6
Letter, *See* Correspondence
Liaison, Commissioned Corps, 77
Manners, dining, 120
Marine Corps, *See*
    U.S. Marine Corps
Medals, wearing of, 23
Meetings, 108
    chairperson, 109
    conventions, 112
    office appointments, 111

parliamentary procedure, 112
participants, 110
Memoranda, *See* Correspondence
Military courtesy and protocol
    address and greeting, 29
    coming to attention, 32
    courtesy, 29
    flag etiquette, 33
    funeral, 36
    handshake, 32
    headgear, 35
    position of honor, 38
    saluting, 39
    ship boarding, 41
    titles, 29
    use of first names, 30
Minority Officers Liaison
    Council, 77
Music Ensemble, 79
Name tag, 17
Navy, *See* U.S. Navy
NOAA Corps, *See*
    U.S. NOAA Corps
Noncommissioned officer, 8
Office of Commissioned Corps
    Force Management, 132
Office of Commissioned Corps
    Operations, 131
Office of Force Readiness
    and Deployment, 84, 131
Office of Public Health
    and Science, 131
Office of Reserve Affairs, 131

Office of Science and
    Communications, 131
Office of the Surgeon
    General, 131, 132
Officer
    aide-de-camp, 64
    chief professional, 68
    color guard, 73
    commissioned, 2, 7
    device standards, 15
    escort, 69
    grades, 7, 8, 12-14
    grooming, 15
    headgear, 16, 35
    insignia, 7, 8, 12-14, 19
    leadership, 4
    line, 8
    noncommissioned, 8
    officership, 2
    personal appearance, 15
    protocol, 82
    qualifications, 7
    ranks, 7, 8, 12-14
    titles, 29-31
    uniform standards, 15
    warrant, 8, 11, 30
Officership, 2
Order of precedence, *See*
    Precedence
Organization
    military services, 143
    U.S. Public Health
        Service, 130

Parliamentary procedure, 112
Place settings, 115
Position of honor, 38
Precedence
    awards and decorations, 20
    ceremonial, official, 49
    guest of honor, 50, 51
    host, 50, 51
    military, 49
    seating arrangements, 51
Presentation ceremony, awards, 53
Presentations and speaking, 94, 103
Professional Advisory
    Committee, 80
Promotion ceremony, 56
Protocol and tradition, 1
Protocol officer, 82
Public Health Service, *See*
    U.S. Public Health Service
Ranks
    commissioned officer,
        7, 8, 12-14
    enlisted personnel, 8-10
    noncommissioned officer, 8
    titles of, 30
    warrant officer, 8, 11
Readiness force, 84
Receiving line, 50
Receptions,
    calls made and paid, 92
    dinners, official, 46
    invitations, 47
    order of precedence, 49

receiving line, 50
Recruiter, 87
Regular Corps, 139
Reserve Corps, 139
Restaurant dining, 124
Retirement ceremony, 59
Ribbons, wearing of, 23
Saluting, 38, 39
Seal
    PHS, 141
    PHS CC, 141
Seating arrangements, 51
Shaking hands, 32
Ship boarding, 41
Speaking, effective, 94, 103
Special duty
    aide-de-camp, 64
    boards, 67
    chief professional officer, 68
    escort officer, 69
    Honor Corps, 73
    Jr Officer Advisory Group, 76
    liaison, CC, 77
    Minority Officers Liaison
        Council, 77
    Music Ensemble, 79
    Professional Advisory
        Committee, 80
    protocol officer, 82
    readiness force, 84
    recruiter, 87
    SG's Policy Advisory
        Council, 88

Surgeon General's Policy
    Advisory Council, 88
Sword, presenting colors, 75
Table manners, 120
Table protocol
    restaurant dining, 124
    table manners, 120
    table settings, 115
Table settings, 115
Telecommunications
    Electronic mail, 105
    Cellular phone, 106
    Telephone, 106
Telephone, 106
Titles
    civilian, 102
    military, 30
Toasts
    dining-out, 45
    dinners, official, 52
    table protocol, 124
Tradition, 1
Travel, 18
Uniformed service
    organizations, 143
Uniforms
    awards and badges, 20, 24
    classifications, 17
    components (chart), 25-28
    considerations, 17
    insignia, 19

medals, 23
name tag, 17
policy, 18
retired officers, 18
ribbons, 23
standards, 15
stars, 23
travel, 18
U.S. Air Force, 145
U.S. Army, 146
U.S. Coast Guard, 147
U.S. Marine Corps, 148
U.S. Navy, 149
U.S. NOAA Corps, 150
U.S. Public Health Service
    agency assignments, 134
    coin, 142
    flag, 141
    history, 139
    march, 142
    mission, 129
    Office of the Surgeon
        General, 131, 132
    organization, 130
    Policy Advisory Council, 88
    Regular Corps, 139
    seal, 141
Warrant officer,
    grades, 8, 11
    qualifications, 8
    titles, 30